中华传统经典养生术
（汉英对照）

(Chinese- English) Traditional and Classical Chinese Health Cultivation

Chief Producer	Li Jie	总策划	李 洁
Chief Compilers	Li Jie Xu Feng Xiao Bin Zhao Xiaoting	总主编	李 洁 许 峰 肖 斌 赵晓霆
Chief Translator	Han Chouping	总主译	韩丑萍
English Language Reviewer	Lawrence Lau	英译主审	劳伦斯·刘

放松功

Fang Song Gong (Relaxation Exercise)

编著 陈昌乐
Compiler Chen Changle

翻译 韩丑萍
Translator Han Chouping

上海科学技术出版社
Shanghai Scientific & Technical Publishers

图书在版编目（CIP）数据

放松功：汉英对照 / 陈昌乐编著；韩丑萍译. —
上海：上海科学技术出版社，2015.5
（中华传统经典养生术）
ISBN 978-7-5478-2562-4

Ⅰ.①放… Ⅱ.①陈… ②韩… Ⅲ.①气功–健身运
动–基本知识–汉、英 Ⅳ.①R214

中国版本图书馆CIP数据核字（2015）第042965号

放松功

编者　陈昌乐

上海世纪出版股份有限公司
上海科学技术出版社　出版

中国图书进出口上海公司　发行

2015年5月第1版
ISBN 978-7-5478-2562-4/R · 880

Fang Song Gong (Relaxation Exercise)

放松功

顾问委员会
Advisory Committee Members

主任

徐建光　陈凯先　严世芸　郑　锦

Directors

Xu Jianguang　Chen Kaixian　Yan Shiyun　Zheng Jin

副主任

施建蓉　胡鸿毅　季　光　张怀琼　余小明　劳力行

Vice Directors

Shi Jianrong　Hu Hongyi　Ji Guang　Zhang Huaiqiong
Yu Xiaoming　Lao Lixing

学术顾问

严世芸　林中鹏　林　欣　李　鼎　俞尔科　王庆其
潘华信　潘华敏　姚玮莉　赵致平　李　磊

Academic Advisers

Yan Shiyun　　Lin Zhongpeng　　Shin Lin　　Li Ding　　Yu Erke
Wang Qingqi　Pan Huaxin　　Pan Huamin　Yao Weili
Zhao Zhiping　Li Lei

Fang Song Gong (Relaxation Exercise) · 放松功

顾问委员会 · Advisory Committee Members

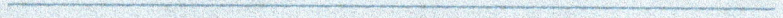

编纂委员会

Compilation Committee Members

总策划

李　洁

Chief Producer

Li Jie

总主编

李　洁　许　峰　肖　斌　赵晓霆

Chief Compilers

Li Jie　Xu Feng　Xiao Bin　Zhao Xiaoting

副总主编

孙　磊　陈昌乐　倪青根

Vice Chief Compilers

Sun Lei　Chen Changle　Ni Qinggen

总主译

韩丑萍

Chief Translator

Han Chouping

副主译

赵海磊

Vice Chief Translator

Zhao Hailei

项目资助

Acknowledgement

· 上海市新闻出版专项扶持资金项目

· 上海市中医药三年行动计划（2015—2018年）"基于〈中华气功史陈列馆〉科普教育基地为核心的〈中医气功文化平台〉建设"
（项目编号：ZY3-WHJS-1-1010）

· Shanghai Press and Publication of special support funds program

· The Three-Year Action Plan for Chinese Medicine in Shanghai (2015–2018) on Construction of Qigong Cultural Platform in the Museum of Chinese Qigong History (Program No: ZY3-WHJS-1-1010)

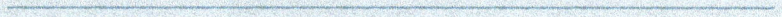

序

Foreword

　　欣闻上海市气功研究所编写的《中华传统经典养生术》丛书即将出版，这是中华原创医学文明传播的一件盛事，特致贺忱。

　　中华传统养生术源远流长，其中导引术更是重要的组成部分，它先于针、灸、药、医而形成，是中华民族最早用以防治疾病、养生保健的重要方法之一。现存早期文献《庄子》《吕氏春秋》《黄帝内经》以及考古发现《引书》《导引图》中均有关于养生导引及其具体方法的记载。此后绵绵数千年的历史长河中，中华养生导引术不断丰富、发展与创新，在自我实践中形成千门万法，在去伪存真中完善理论体系。20世纪后叶，古之导引术又以现代"气功"的面目再次席卷中华大地，并享誉海内外。时至今天，中华导引术仍然以其"人天合一"的整体观思想与丰富多姿的养生导引方法独立于世界自然医药之林，滋润着人类身心世界。事实表明，中华导引术已经形成为一门博大精深的学术体系。它所研究的是人之物质基础（精）与自组织能力（神）相互关系的规律，是关于"人"——这个地球上最复杂系统达到和谐与协调的一门学问。

　　我和上海市气功研究所相识逾30年，该所自20世纪70年代的中医研究所开始，气功与导引就是关注、研究的重点领域；80年代中期更名气功研究所后，更是全力着眼于现代气功的研究与中华导引术的弘扬。《中华传统经典养生术》是上海市气功研究所多年来所教授养生导引术、气功功法的汇编与总结，对于帮助学习、普及推广现代导引术具有较好的价值。希望此丛书的出版，能够进一步带动当前养生导引术在海内外的健康发展，推动中华优秀文化走向世界各地。

　　是以为序。

林中鹏

2015年3月

It is with great pleasure that I learn the *Traditional and Classical Chinese Health Cultivation* series compiled by the Shanghai Qigong Research Institute will be published soon. This means a lot to the spread of Chinese medical civilization.

Traditional Chinese health cultivation has a long-standing and well-established history. As an important part of health cultivation practice, Dao Yin exercise was used for disease prevention and treatment as well as life cultivation before acupuncture, moxibustion and herbal medicine. The recordings of *Dao Yin* and its specific exercise methods can be traced back to the *Zhuangzi, Lü Shi Chun Qiu* (The Annals of Lü Buwei), *Huang Di Nei Jing* (the Yellow Emperor's Inner Classic) and archaeologically unearthed books such as *Yin Shu* (a book on Dao Yin) and *Dao Yin Tu* (Dao Yin Diagram). After this, the thousands of years have witnessed the enrichment, progress and innovation of Chinese *Dao Yin* practice, coupled with emergence of numerous methods and perfection of its theoretical system. In late 20th century, the ancient *Dao Yin* exercise became exceptionally popular across China in the form of 'qigong'. Today, Chinese *Dao Yin* exercise remains flourish with its holistic 'Man-Nature Unity' idea and various exercise methods that benefit both body and mind. Facts show that there is a profound academic system behind Chinese *Dao Yin* exercise. This system studies the interactions between material foundation (essence) and self-organization ability (mind). In other words, it studies the way to achieve harmony and coordination of human being—the most complex system on earth.

I've established a friendship with the Shanghai Qigong Research Institute for 30 years. Ever since its founding in 1970s as a Research Institute of Chinese Medicine, qigong and *Dao Yin* have always been the research priorities of the Institute. The focuses on qigong and *Dao Yin* have been more highlighted in 1980s when the Institute was renamed as a Qigong Research Institute. I firmly believe that the

Traditional and Classical Chinese Health Cultivation series are of great significance in popularizing modern *Dao Yin* exercise. I sincerely wish the book series can further promote *Dao Yin* exercise at home and abroad and spread excellent Chinese culture.

For this, I wrote this forward.

Lin Zhongpeng

March 2015

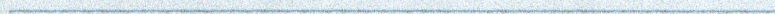

前 言

气 以 臻 道

农历乙未早春,正是上海市气功研究所创建三十周年之际,恰逢气功学术发展枯木迎春之季。在此,我们谨向海内外气功学界发出倡言——构建现代气功"气以臻道"的学术思想。

所谓"气以臻道",首先是指气功学术发展必须树立一个大方向,即中华传统文化精神的最高目标——"道";其次是指通过对"气"的感性体验与理性认知,使生命更趋向"道",与"道"合一。道者,规律、目标也;气者,方法、途径也;臻者,趋向、完善也。气-道共同构成"气以臻道"学术思想内核。其中气为实、主行,是具体之指;道为虚、主理,是抽象之喻。气因道而展,道由气而实;气以道归,道以气显;气借道而实际指归,道假气而理性论证。气功学术发展必须气、道并重,互印互证,理行一贯。两者既各尽其责、各擅其能,又有主从之别。"道"因标指形上本体而为万法归宗之源;"气"每描述形下万法而成法法生灭之流。"道"经思维抽象提炼,揭示规律、规则之理性思辨;"气"常直叙主观感觉,表述体会、觉受的感性认识。道-气,一主一从,一虚一实,构成中华气功学术思想的本质内涵。

"气以臻道"学术思想之主体是"道",是指向真理之道路,是学术文化人文精神的体现,也是先人用身心去实践生命运化规律的心得体验,古人称为"内证之学"。"道"的外延旁及"功"和"术",可以包括各种神秘现象、气功现象、特异现象,古人称为"神通法术"。当今,现代科学研究介入传统气功学术是时代进步的表现,它为我们观察生命奥秘打开了一个全新的视角。透过唯象的研究,重新激发起人类对生命的思考与敬重,重新挖掘出科技文明下的人文精神,而非单纯地将生命物质化,这才是现代科学介入传统气功的人文价值所在。

有鉴于此，我们倡议构建现代气功研究之 "气以臻道" 学术思想，让中华传统文化与现代科学携起手来，揭示生命真谛，回归大道本源。

上海市气功研究所
2015年春

Advocacy for *Qi-Dao Harmony* in Modern Qigong Practice

The year 2015 is a Chinese new year of yin wood sheep (*Yi Wei* in Chinese). Wood, in Chinese culture on five elements (*Wu Xing*), is connected to the season of spring. The year 2015 also marks the 30th anniversary of the founding of Shanghai Qigong Research Institute. With a strong belief that the spring of 2015 will bring new hope to qigong study, we hereby advocate the concept of 'Qi-*Dao Harmony*' for its academic advance.

The term *Qi-Dao Harmony* has two underlying implications. First, it implies that *dao* is the ultimate goal of traditional Chinese culture and the general orientation for academic qigong advance. Second, it implies that our lives shall combine into one with the *dao* through perception and understanding of qi. In summary, this term means to achieve and perfect *dao* through qi exercise. The 'qi' here is weighted and refers to practice. The '*dao*' here is unweighted and refers to principles. Without *dao*, qi cannot extend; without qi, *dao* cannot become weighted. Qi finds its origin in *dao* and *dao* manifests itself in qi. Qi returns to *dao* eventually and *dao* supports qi theoretically. It's essential for people in academic qigong field to pay equal attention to qi and *dao*. The two have a principal-subordinate relationship. The metaphysical *dao* is the origin of all methods. The physical qi is the practice of all methods. *Dao* is about the abstract thinking and reveals the laws and rules. Qi is about the subjective feelings and tells experience and perception. Qi and *dao* constitute the essence of academic idea in Chinese qigong.

Let's get a deeper look into the concept of *Qi-Dao Harmony*. Also known as the 'learning of internal evidence', *dao* is the way to truth. It contains humanistic spirit and physical and mental experience of our ancestors. *Dao* extends to exercise (*gong*) and a variety of magic arts including mysterious, qigong and extrasensory phenomena. Today, modern scientific qigong research offers a new insight into the mysteries of life. The phenomenological research rekindles our reflection and respect towards life and enables us to re-discover humanism from modern civilization greatly impacted by science and technology. This is the real value of scientific research on traditional qigong in this materialized world.

To this end, we advocate the academic concept of '*Qi-Dao Harmony*' in modern qigong research. We believe the combination of traditional Chinese culture and modern science can help us to reveal the truth of life and return to the origin of the great *dao*.

Shanghai Qigong Research Institute
Spring 2015

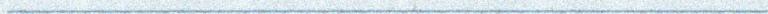

编写说明

Words from the Compilers

中华传统养生术根植于中国传统哲学、中医学和养生学，是人体自我身心锻炼的有效方法。

随着倡导"主动健康"概念日益深入人心，具有调身、调息、调心功能的中华传统养生术，以其传统的养修理论、独特的身心效果蜚声海内外，引起世人的广泛关注。但近期国内外少见中国传统养生术的书籍出版，尤其没有成套、成系列的经典养生类作品问世，更缺乏英汉对照的专业著作。

上海中医药大学上海市气功研究所研究人员在前期研究工作基础上，精选中华传统经典养生术共八种，从历史源流、功法理论、特色要领、图解动作、分解说明与具体运用几方面进行中文编纂，由上海中医药大学中医英语专业人员进行翻译。并邀请专家进行中文审稿，邀请美国友三中医药大学Lawrence Lau先生审定英文翻译。

本套丛书详细地将八种中华经典养生术以图文并茂、视频摄像的形式记录下来，配以光盘，非常方便学习与传播，尤其便于海外养生爱好者以英语来学习。

本套丛书编纂过程中，得到上海市中医药三年行动计划（2015—2018年）"基于〈中华气功史陈列馆〉科普教育基地为核心的〈中医气功文化平台〉建设"（项目编号：ZY3-WHJS-1-1010）资助。

编者

Traditional Chinese health cultivation includes a variety of body-mind exercises, which are deeply rooted in ancient Chinese philosophy and medicine.

Today, the concept of 'health initiative (an ability to achieve physical, mental and social well-being)' has become well recognized.

Traditional Chinese health cultivation exercises are attracting worldwide attention because of their unique effects in regulating the breathing, body and mind. However, there are few books in this regard, especially the classical book series. There are even fewer bilingual Chinese-English versions of these books.

Based on their previous studies, research staff at the Shanghai Qigong Research Institute compiled eight traditional and classical health cultivation exercise methods, covering their history, theoretical foundation, characteristics and key principles, illustrated movements and application. Then these contents have been translated by professional interpreters at Shanghai University of Traditional Chinese Medicine. The Chinese version was reviewed by an expert team. The English version was reviewed by Dr. Lawrence Lau at the Yo San University of Traditional Chinese Medicine.

In addition to illustrations and videos are also available for readers, especially overseas health cultivation fans to learn.

This books series have been funded by the Three-Year Action Plan for Chinese Medicine in Shanghai (2015-2018) on Construction of Qigong Cultural Platform in the Museum of Chinese Qigong History (Program No: ZY3–WHJS–1–1010).

Compilers

目 录

Table of Contents

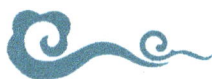

放　松　功　　•　　*Fang Song Gong* (Relaxation Exercise)

History

源
流

放松功是通过自身的主动调节,逐渐使身体、呼吸、心理放松下来,达到三调合一境界的一组气功功法,也是练好其他气功功法的基础功法。

Fang Song Gong serves as the foundation of many other qigong exercises. It aims to relax the body, breathing and mind through active regulation, eventually achieving the unity of three regulations.

放松法由来已久,千百年来,在与自然的搏斗中,紧张、疲劳一直困扰着人们,为了更好地休息,保养身心,人们不断地寻求着各种放松的方法。虽然古人没有直接说"放松"这两个字,但从文献中,我们可以发现大量可以借鉴的方法。

Over the past thousands of years, people have always been experiencing fatigue and tension during their struggle for survival. As a result, they have never stopped seeking relaxation methods for better rest and wellness. Although ancient Chinese people never mentioned the term *Fang Song* (relaxation), we found numerous methods from ancient literature.

例如《素问·移精变气论》中论述:"内无眷慕之累,外无伸官之形,此恬惔之世,邪不能深入也。"告诉我们放松心理的内容和作用,内心不受七情干扰,外形不受名利驱使等奔波劳碌,保持安静愉快淡泊的心态,不容易遭到病邪侵害。

The *Su Wen Yi Jing Bian Qi Lun* (chapter 13 of the Basic Questions) states, 'Internally, you are not disturbed by seven emotions. Externally, you are not bothered by fame and wealth.

With such a peaceful mind, there's no way for exogenous pathogenic factors to attack you'.

《素问·上古天真论》曰:"余闻上古有真人者,提挈天地,把握阴阳。呼吸精气,独立守神,肌肉若一,故能寿敝天地,无有终时。此其道生。"告诉我们在生活中要顺应自然规律,练功时要调节精神内守,浑身肌肉要协调一致,长时间练习,就可以达到延长寿命的效果。这些操作方法,是放松功的操作要点。

The *Su Wen Shang Gu Tian Zhen Lun* (chapter 1 of the Basic Questions) states, 'Sages in antiquity follow the law of yin and yang, exercise breathing, concentrate their mind, and coordinate body muscles. Therefore they can achieve health and longevity'.

《庄子·大宗师》记载了孔子与颜回的对话,"何谓坐忘?"颜回曰:"堕肢体,黜聪明,离形去知,同于大通,此谓坐忘。"提示静坐的时候不要过分关注肢体,也不要去思考问题,要排除杂念,逐渐就可以进入到一种祥和、平静的状态。这里的操作和放松功已经非常接近了,可以说已经具备了放松功静功的雏形。

The *Zhuang Zi Da Zong Shi* (Inner chapter 6 of Zhuangzi) recorded the dialogue between Confucius and his disciple Yan Hui. 'What do you mean by sitting and forgetting everything?' Yan Hui replied, 'My connection with the body and its parts is dissolved; my perceptive organs are discarded. Thus leaving my material form, and bidding farewell to my knowledge, I become one with the Great Pervader. This I call sitting and forgetting all things'.

《神仙食气金匮妙录》中也提道: 存想自己衣被皆去,骨节

皆解,自觉运行体中,经营周身等。讲述了放松过程中的内在操作,即自我感觉性操作,对我们今天练放松功的心理操作仍然具有很强的指导意义。

The *Shen Xian Shi Qi Jin Kui Miao Lu* (Wonderful Recordings of Golden Chamber on Ingestion of Qi by Immortals) also mentioned the self-perceptive exercise: visualize your clothes and quilts are removed, your bones and joints are dissolved and qi circulates freely through your body.

《童蒙止观》一书中对练功时的呼吸做了较为详细的描述,"坐时息虽无声,而出入结滞不通,是喘相也。云何气相? 坐时息虽无声,亦不结滞,而出入不细,是气相也。云何息相? 不声,不结,不粗,出入绵绵,若存若亡,资神安隐,情抱悦豫。此是息相也。"指出了练功时正确的呼吸方式,和其表现形式。只有出入绵绵、若存若亡地呼吸,才有益于进入高层次气功境界。这种"息相"的呼吸形式正是放松功中运用的呼吸形式。

The *Tong Meng Zhi Guan* (Samatha-vipasyana or Insight Meditation) described the breathing during qigong practice in detail, 'Wind phase refers to raspy and noisy breathing through the nose; gasp phase refers to restricted or choppy breathing; qi phase refers to rough breathing and quiescent phase refers to fine and deep breathing'. This clearly states that the quiescent phase can help you enter a qigong state.

《太清调气经》中的委身法对练功时身体的感觉做了生动的描述:"候四体清和,内无思念,行止寝卧而调其息,凝然委身,如委其衣,以置于榻。无筋无骨,无神无识,纵身纵心,如彼委衣,寂寂沉沉,放其身体,澄神炼气,即百节开张,筋脉畅通,津液注流。"讲述了放松过程中身心的操作,身体轻松,内心平和,心无杂念,呼吸调匀,四肢自然垂下,感觉好像没有了筋骨,没有了意识,坚持这样练习,精神会更加清爽。

The *Tai Qing Tiao Qi Jing* (Supreme Clarity Method on Qi Regulation) also vividly described the physical feelings during qigong practice, 'When your body relaxed and your mind calmed down (with no distracting thoughts), your breathing slows down and your limbs loosen up. Little by little, you felt like the sinews and bones are dissolved and your consciousness is gone. With this, your qi and blood can flow freely throughout your body and you feel more refreshed'.

近代人丁福保在1943年写的《最真确之健康长寿法》一书中也介绍了与放松功相似的"弛缓法":取仰卧式,轻轻合眼,感安静后,想及自己之两眼已轻闭,头额弛缓,颜面亦全然轻松,齿在口中若有若无;又思及自己之手足也同样轻松安放,心脏之鼓动安静而松弛,呼吸轻松而自如,腹部也全部松弛,有如溶化,全然不为何物所拘束。松弛又分表面的松,即先使头盖、颜面、颈、胸、腹、背、手足之骨骼筋肉组织放松;而后及于深达于心脏、血管、细胞、胃肠及内分泌腺等,用以治病。这种从头到脚依次放松的方法后来发展成为放松功中的分段放松法。

Ding Fu-bao (1874-1952) introduced a similar relaxation exercise in the *Most Correct Method for Health and Longevity* (printed in 1943): Take a supine lying position and gently close the eyes. After a while, visualize the forehead and face loosened up, the teeth are sometimes there but sometimes not; then visualize the hands and feet relaxed, then the heart, breathing and abdomen, feeling like they are all dissolved. Evidently, relaxation starts from the surface of the body — skull, face, neck, chest, abdomen, back, hands and feet, and then goes deeper — the heart, vessels, cells, intestines, stomach and endocrine gland. This exercise later became segmental relaxation method in *Fang Song Gong*.

20世纪上海市气功研究所的专家在总结前人经验的基础上，结合自身练功经验和教功体会，创编出一组通过对身体姿势、动作、呼吸、心理的主动调节，解除紧张，消除疲劳，使身心逐渐放松，进入轻松、自然、舒适状态的一组方法，并命名为放松功。

In the 20th century, experts at the Shanghai Qigong Research Institute compiled a set of methods to actively regulate the body posture, movements, breathing and mental activities. These methods are named *Fang Song Gong*. Practicing *Fang Song Gong* can relieve stress and fatigue and relax the body and mind.

在20世纪五六十年代，放松功作为南方功法的代表与北方的内养功一起在实践、教学、科研等方面做了大量工作，并称气功界的"南北双璧"。在随后的几十年里，放松功被广泛地应用于临床，并取得诸多成果，尤其是在防治高血压病方面最为突出。由上海市高血压病研究所牵头进行的相关实验持续了30年，发表数十篇论文，证明习练放松功对高血压患者有辅助治疗作用，长期习练放松功有助于控制血压，并可以预防并发症的出现。

In 1950s and 1960s, *Fang Song Gong* from the South of China and *Nei Yang Gong* from the North of China were known as 'double jade' for their involvement in practice, education and scientific research. In the decades that followed, *Fang Song Gong* has been extensively used in clinical practice and proven especially effective for the prevention and treatment of hypertension. Scholars at the Shanghai Hypertension Research Institute conducted 30 years of clinical trials and published dozens of papers regarding the effect of *Fang Song Gong* on hypertension. Clinical studies have suggested that practice of *Fang Song Gong* has supportive therapeutic efficacy, long-time practice can help to control blood pressure and prevent complications.

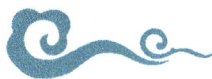

放 松 功 · *Fang Song Gong* (Relaxation Exercise)

Theoretical Foundation

理论基础

以中医理论为基础
Chinese Medical Theory

放松功有很多放松方法，下面以三线放松功为例讲述其理论基础。三线放松功的功法理论来源于中医理论，尤其是经络学说。例如，三线放松法吸收了经络学的理论，从上向下沿身体的前面、侧面、后面依次放松，这些区域也正是身体重要经络循行经过的地方。身体前面大部分属于足阳明胃经和任脉，胸腹部还有足太阴脾经、足厥阴肝经和足少阴肾经循行；头部侧面属于手少阳三焦经和足少阳经胆经；两臂经络丰富，手三阳经、三阴经都分布于上肢；身体后面属于足太阳膀胱经和督脉。这三条放松线路，涵盖了身体十二正经和任督二脉。

Fang Song Gong originated from Chinese medical theory, especially the meridian theory. For example, the three-line relaxation method follows the anterior, lateral and posterior aspects of the body, where are also the pathways of different meridians. More specifically, stomach and Ren meridians travel in the anterior aspect of the body, spleen, liver and kidney meridians also travel in the chest and abdominal area. *Sanjiao* and gallbladder meridians travel in the lateral aspect of the body. Three-yang and three-yin meridians of the hand travel along the upper limbs. Bladder and Du meridians travel in the posterior aspect of the body. The three relaxation lines cover all twelve regular meridians and two extraordinary meridians (Du and Ren).

《黄帝内经灵枢·经脉》说："经脉者，所以决死生，处百病，调虚实,不可不通。"可见经络在人体的重要性。每条放松线路的止息点都是井穴,井穴是经脉气血的起源,最后的止息点也都是身体重要穴位。意守这些穴位,对身体气血运行都有着显著的调节作用。在做拍打放松功时,叩击的部位也大多是身体的重要穴位,这些穴位都是人体气血汇聚的重要场所,轻轻地叩击,具有激发经气的作用。放松功正是通过放松身体、呼吸、心理来调节人体的经络气血,进而促进健康,消除疾病的。

The *Huang Di Nei Jing* (Yellow Emperor's Internal Classic) states, 'Since meridians can decide life or death, ailments and deficiency or excess conditions can be regulated through meridians, they have to be unobstructed'. The end points of each line are Jing-well points, located at the on the fingers and toes of the four extremities where qi of meridians emerges. Focusing mental consciousness on these points can help with circulation of qi and blood. In tapping relaxation method, important points (where qi and blood gather) are tapped to activate meridian qi. By relaxing the body, breathing and mind, *Fang Song Gong* regulates meridian qi and blood, promotes health and eliminates illnesses.

放松是手段与目的的结合

Relaxation is a means, process and end

放松是一种手段,一个过程,也是一种状态。

放松作为一种手段,是因为它可以作为一种操作方法来帮助我们放松。例如身体紧张时,我们把身体分成前面、侧面、后面三条线,或者把身体分成若干段,这样化整为零,就便于操作了;呼吸急促时我们逐渐地延长呼吸,使呼吸变得又细又长,均匀柔和;心理抑郁、焦虑时我们把意念略微集中一下,在呼气时默念"松……"并轻轻地听自己发出的声音,随着声音逐渐减轻，我们的内心也会逐渐平静下来。

Relaxation can be a means to relax. For example, physical stress can be relieved along the three (anterior, lateral and posterior) lines or by segments. In case of rapid breathing, you can adjust your breathing to be fine, long, even and soft. In case of mental depression or anxiety, you can concentrate your mind, aspirate the sound 'Song', listen to your sound and gradually calm down.

放松作为一个过程，是因为从开始放松到真的松下来需要一段时间，不可能一蹴而就。习练放松功时，会发现放松是有层次的，随着放松程度的加深，会逐渐感知到不同的紧张，而且，身体、呼吸、意念在放松过程中也是相互制约、相互促进的。随着放松程度的深入，很多开始感觉放松的部位还不够放松，甚至会感到紧张，但这时的紧张已不像最初那样明显，而是比较细微了。于是开始新一轮的放松，就这样几经反复，放松的层次也会逐渐深入。所以要练好放松功，做到松透，绝非一日之功。

Relaxation can be a process, because it cannot be achieved overnight. When practicing *Fang Song Gong*, you can find relaxation has different levels. Along with relaxation, you can also encounter new tension. In addition, body, breathing and mind can supplement and inhibit one another. Along with further relaxation, you may feel the relaxed areas are not relaxed enough; you may even feel tension in a delicate way. Then you move on to next round or level of relaxation.

放松作为一种状态，是因为它具有一定的生理、心理特征。在身体上表现为，姿势中正安舒、动作轻盈灵活；呼吸上表现为深、长、柔、细；心理上表现为平和内敛、恬淡虚无等。

Relaxation can be a psychological or physiological state.

Physically, relaxation can manifest as upright, comfortable, lively and agile body as well as deep, long, soft and fine breathing. Psychologically, relaxation manifests as a peaceful, tranquil mind.

三调合一

Unity of Three Regulations

"三调合一"是指随着练功境界的提高，在感觉上动作、呼吸、心理三者之间的界限逐渐模糊，最终三者融为一体的气功状态。这时我们也不再单独的调整动作、呼吸或心理，而是把他们作为一个整体来调整。"三调合一"是气功锻炼的本质特征，放松功也不例外。

As an essential characteristic of qigong practice, unity of three regulations is a high-level qigong state. During this state, there are no clear boundaries between body movements, breathing and mental consciousness.

调身：是调控身体静止或运动状态的操作活动，也称"炼形""身法"等。习练放松功可以选用的姿势较多，有站、坐、卧、行四种，练功时可以根据每个人的体质、需求来选取适合的姿势。具体内容将在后面详细介绍。调身的意义在于使身体的状态与练功所要求的境界相应。练松通法、三线放松法、分段放松法、局部放松法、整体放松法和倒行放松法等偏于静功的功法时，调身使身体保持一个相对固定的姿势，有助于气血运行，有利于进入呼吸柔顺、内心平静的气功境界。如果身体偏斜甚至扭曲，或某一部分处于紧张状态，难以放松，那么，这些地方的气血运行也会受到一定影响，在放松路线经过这些部位时，呼吸也难以做到深、长、柔、细，心理也会有相应变化；而练振颤放松法和拍打放松法等偏于动功的功法时，调身表现为动作轻松、舒缓与整体协调性，有助于调整气血运行，有利于调节脏腑功能，如果某处紧张，难以放松，会表为抖动时不协调、拍打时会有酸麻痛胀等感觉。

Regulating the body means to adjust static posture or dynamic body movements. It aims to match physical state with qigong realm. As for static exercises including Relaxing and Unblocking Method, Three-line Relaxation Method, Segmental Relaxation Method, Local Relaxation Method, Whole Body Relaxation Method and Reversed Relaxation Method, regulating the body can help with a fixed body posture to allow smooth flow of qi and blood and enter a qigong state with even breathing and tranquil mind. Deviated or twisted body position or tension in certain body parts can obstruct flow of qi and blood along the relaxation lines, further affecting the breathing and mind. As for dynamic exercises including Shaking/Trembling and Tapping Relaxation Methods, regulating the body can coordinate gentle slow movements to allow smooth circulation of qi and blood and benefit functions of the zang-fu organs. Tension in certain body parts can cause uncoordinated trembling; you may feel pain, numbness, soreness and dissension upon tapping.

调息：是调控呼吸的操作活动，也称"炼气"，又称"呼吸""吐纳"等。调息的意义在于通过调控呼吸而孕育和引导内气，这是进入气功境界的重要操作环节。呼吸与内气直接相关，通常练功过程中随着日常呼吸的逐渐减弱，内气的活动逐渐加强。一吸一呼为一息，其中尤以呼气与内气密切相关，内气多随呼气运行，故放松功注重于调控呼气。现代研究已证明，调息可调节自主神经系统中交感神经和副交感神经的张力，从而可以调整相应的内脏组织器官的功能。其中呼气时副交感神经兴奋,更有利于放松。习练松通法、三线放松法、分段放松法、局部放松法、整体放松法和倒行放松法等偏于静功的功法时,在呼气同时配合默念"松……"吐气要均匀缓慢,不要急促。发音时要放松身心,重在放松的意念和感觉,而不在发出的声音上。开始时,为集中精力,发音相对较为清楚,随着放松程度的加深,意识活动逐渐减少,声音会越来越轻,甚至有些模糊,逐渐只剩下"ong"的音,最后只剩下"ong"字的感觉,已经听不到任何声音。这时的呼吸已经由平日里粗重、散乱的呼吸逐步调整到了深透、缓慢、细长、均匀的呼吸状态;内心也会进入平静、无我的状态。练振颤放松法时,操作要点是呼吸自然,与振颤或抖动的频率协调一致;练拍打放松法时同样注重呼气,操作要点是在呼气时叩击身体,吸气时不要叩击身体。姿势中正自然时,气血运行容易通畅,身体也容易放松。

Regulating the breathing means to adjust your inhalation and exhalation. It aims to cultivate and guide internal qi and help you enter a qigong state. Breathing is directly associated with internal qi. Along with gradual decrease of everyday breathing, internal qi may gradually increase. Since internal qi is particularly associated with exhalation, Fang Song Gong mainly stresses on regulating exhalation. Modern studies have proven that breathing regulation can adjust sympathetic and parasympathetic tension and thus benefit functions of internal organs. Exhalation can activate parasympathetic nerve and help to relax. As for static exercises including Relaxing and Unblocking Method, Three-line Relaxation Method, Segmental Relaxation Method, Local Relaxation Method, Whole Body Relaxation Method and Reversed Relaxation Method, aspirate the sound of 'Song' during even slow exhalation. While aspirating the sound of 'Song', place the focus on relaxing the body and mind instead of the sound itself. At the beginning, aspirate the sound clearly to concentrate the mind. Over time, along with decreased mental activities, aspirate the sound more gently and vaguely, like the sound of 'ong'. By now, the rough scattered breathing has become deep, slow, long, fine and even, followed by a tranquil no-self mental state. As for shaking/trembling relaxation method, it's essential to breath naturally to coordinate the frequency of trembling or shaking. As for tapping relaxation method, it's also essential to tap the body during exhalation only. An upright comfortable body posture can help with smooth circulation of qi and blood as well as relaxation of the body.

调心：是调控心理状态的操作活动，也称"炼神""炼己"等。调心的意义在于改变日常意识活动的内容和方式，是进入气功境界所需要的意识状态。一般日常生活中的意识活动属外向性，练气功则需要将意识活动转为内向，进而导致意识活动内容和方式的变化。习练松通法、三线放松法、分段放松法、局部放松法、整体放松法和倒行放松法等偏于静功的功法时，调心是三调中的主导因素，在我们意守一个的部位时，该处的气机就会得到调整，气机调畅了，姿势也就变得中正安舒了，呼吸也就容易达到深、长、柔、细了。古人说"形不正则气不顺，气不顺则意不宁，意不宁则神散乱"，就是这个道理。

Regulating the mind means to adjust mental activities. It aims to alter the content and model of daily consciousness and help you enter a qigong state. It's necessary to shift from extroversion in daily living to introversion in qigong practice, and further change the content and model of daily consciousness. As for static exercises including Relaxing and Unblocking Method, Three-line Relaxation Method, Segmental Relaxation Method, Local Relaxation Method, Whole Body Relaxation Method and Reversed Relaxation Method, regulating the mind is the leading factor among three regulations. When you place our mental consciousness on a specific body part, qi activity in that body part can be regulated. Subsequently, your body can become upright and your breathing can be deep, long, soft and fine. Just as the saying goes, 'Without an upright body, there will be no free flow of qi; with free flow of qi, there will be no tranquility of mind; without tranquility of mind, there will be disordered spirit'.

三调之间有着密切的关系,相互影响,相互制约,相互促进。不仅是身体紧张放不松会影响呼吸和心理,呼吸急促也会导致身体和心理的紧张,而心理紧张同样也会导致身体的紧张和呼吸节律的紊乱。所以放松功同时涉及身体、呼吸、心理三个方面,在习练时可以从任何一个方面入手,通过这个方面带动另外两个方面,最终的目标都是三者协调一致,融为一体,我们称之为三调合一。

Three regulations are closely connected and can affect one another. Physical stress can affect breathing and mind. Rapid breathing can cause physical and mental stress. And mental stress can disturb breathing and cause body tension. *Fang Song Gong* involves all three aspects — the body, breathing and mind. Exercise from each aspect can positively influence the other two aspects. The ultimate goal is unity of three regulations.

松紧有度
Combination of Relaxation and Intension

"松"和"紧"是一对矛盾,放松功中两者是辩证统一。
Relaxation and intension are unity of opposites.

首先,在练功的过程中松中有紧,紧中有松。习练放松功时不是要身体瘫软下来，因为瘫软的身体，看似放松，却有很多关节受到挤压，即使平躺在床上，彻底瘫软的身体也不利于气血的运行。所以练功时的松是在机体保持一定张力下的松，古人称之为"松而不懈"；同样道理，放松功的坐式与站式，都要求"正"，看似要求身体收紧，其实不然，这里"正"是放松后气血充盈的自然端正，如同树木在阳光、水分充足的情况下，茂盛的生长时，呈现出的舒展条达。不是像木偶一样，刻板的僵直的姿势，古人称之为"紧而不僵"。

First, *Fong Song Gong* exercise requires unity of intension and relaxation. Relaxation does not mean flaccidity. Flaccidity of the body may squeeze multiple joints. Even in a lying position, qi and blood cannot flow freely in a completely flaccid body. Relaxation in qigong practice is not sluggish. Likewise, an upright body is essential for *Fang Song Gong* in either sitting or standing. However, upright is not stiff or rigid. The 'upright' here is a relaxed state with abundance of qi and blood, just like exuberant growth of trees with sufficient water and sunlight.

其次，在放松的过程中，松和紧是相互促进、相互转化的。在练放松功时，把意识集中在某处，叫做意守，意守是现代气功常用术语。意，指意识、意念或精神。守，指集中和保持住。意守通常是指气功锻炼过程中，将意念集中和保持在身体某一部位，或某一事物上的方法和过程。例如：习练三线放松功时，完整习练一遍，有27个部位，三个止息点，和下丹田，共31个意守部位。意守的过程就是紧的过程，通过紧来促进放松，可以帮助排除杂念，实现"一念代万念"，逐步达到气功放松入静的状态，并在此基础上体察身体各方面的感觉与变化，进行自我调整，以取得更好的练功效果。在习练松通法、三线放松法、分段放松法、局部放松法、整体放松法和倒行放松法等偏于静功的功法时，意守一个部位，默念"松"字，就是从紧到松的过程。再如，练振颤放松法和拍打放松法时，拍打是紧的过程，通过拍打的紧，可以使身体放松。

Second, relaxation and intension support and transform into each other. During *Fang Song Gong* practice, you need to focus your mental consciousness on certain body parts or things. This process of intension can help to relax the body, remove distracting thoughts, 'replace ten thousand thoughts with one thought', and gradually enters tranquility. Over time, you can improve your exercise result through continuous experience and self-adjustment. As for static exercises including Relaxing and Unblocking Method, Three-line Relaxation Method, Segmental Relaxation Method, Local Relaxation Method, Whole Body Relaxation Method and Reversed Relaxation Method, focus your consciousness on one body part and aspirate the sound of 'Song' in silence. This is a process from intension to relaxation. As for Shaking/Trembling and Tapping Relaxation Methods, the body is relaxed through shaking, trembling or tapping.

循序渐进

Practice Step by Step

放松本身又可分为不同的层次，在这里我们大致分为三个阶段：松静阶段，松通阶段，松空阶段。放松的程度层次，包括身体和心理两方面，而这两个方面又是相互关联的。首先，身体的放松有利于心理的放松，而要做到身体放松，除了摆好姿势以外，还需要一定的心理活动的参与，意念不足，放松欠佳，意念过重，本身又会造成精神紧张，也不利于放松。所以，对于每一位练功者来讲，要根据练功过程中的自我感受，做出适当的自我调整，逐步达到"松"的要求。

There are three levels of relaxation, namely relaxation

and tranquility, relaxation and unblocking, and relaxation and emptiness. Each level of relaxation involves the body and mind. Your mind tends to quiet down when your body is loosened up. To loosen up your body, you need posture adjustment as well as mental activities. Without mental consciousness, you cannot relax the body completely. However, excessive mental consciousness may cause new stress or tension. Consequently, it's important to adjust in accordance with individual experience and achieve 'relaxation'.

开始习练放松功的要求是身体松弛,内心平静状态即可,即感到周身上下、躯体内外及肢节皮毛舒松自然,气血运行通畅,排除杂念,内心平静,这就标志着习练者进入了松静阶段。进一步坚持练功,会感觉到身体逐渐松开,有的人是一层一层松开,有的人是一块一块松开,放松感在体内逐渐弥漫开来扩散到每一个角落。有的人感觉像坐在水中,有的人感觉自己像冰块一样融化,有的人感觉自己肌体与骨架在慢慢分离,渐渐地仅剩下一副骨架,其余部分均被溶解,甚至仅存的骨架也被溶解,整个身心处在一种若有若无、时隐时现的状态。这些都是气血通畅的表现,所以叫松通阶段,这时心理更加平静,并有种说不出的喜悦。最后进入松空阶段,这个阶段的表现以空无为主要特征,这时连若隐若现的身体也消失了,内心也会超越平静,进入一种空无的状态,需要说明的是这种空无不是真空,不是完全寂静,而是一种生动活泼的虚空状态,这时的呼吸已经十分缓慢细微,如果继续坚持练功,最终可以达到三调合一的境界。对于初学者来说,达到松静阶段的要求就可以了,后面的松通、松空阶段,只可顺其自然,不能着意追求,否则,会欲速则不达。

For beginners of *Fang Song Gong*, it's essential to have a relaxed body (with free flow of qi and blood) and a peaceful mind (no distracting thoughts). This is the level of relaxation and tranquility. Over time, you can feel your body is gradually loosened up layer by layer or piece by piece. Little by little, the relaxation feeling spread to every corner from inside the body. This is the level of relaxation and unblocking (unobstructed flow of qi and blood). In this level, people may have various feelings and experience joy beyond words. Some feel like sitting in water. Some fee like a piece of melting ice. Some feel like the body is being separated from the skeleton, then the other parts of the body is dissolved except for the skeleton, gradually the skeleton is also dissolved and the body becomes vague. The final level is relaxation and emptiness. In this level, even the vague body disappeared and you enter an empty state of mind. The 'empty' here is not vacuum or entire silence but lively and vigorous. In this state, your breathing becomes slow and fine. Further practice can lead you to unity of three regulations. It's sufficient for beginners to reach the first level. As for the last two levels, just flow through it and do not force yourself to pursue, just like the saying goes, more haste, less speed.

三因制宜

Practice according to individual age, gender and constitution

　　关于练功的姿势因个人的体质不同，身体状况不同，放松的姿势也会略有差别。例如患有肩周炎的人，患侧上肢难以放松，很难做到虚腋；膝关节损伤的人，患侧膝关节受力程度差，重心常常向健侧偏移，这些都是正常现象。在放松深入到一定层次后，身体会逐渐找到最适合自己当下的姿势，呼吸也会找到最适合的频率，由于身体的状况不同，这是的状态也不尽相同，达到"只求神意足，不求形骸似"的境界即可。要点是找到最适合自己放松的状态，而不是千篇一律的追求过分的中正，那样会适得其反，造成紧张。

Relaxation posture varies from person to person. For example, it's difficult for people with frozen shoulder to relax the upper limbs and armpits; and it's natural for people with knee joint injury to shift the body weight to the healthy side. Over time, you will find the most suitable body posture and breathing frequency for you. You do not have to be too fastidious about an 'upright' posture.

关于练功量，每个人的体质状况不同，耐受力不一样，尤其对于患者而言，尚有虚实之变化，所以，要针对不同的个体制定合理的练功量。练功量过大，疏泄太过，易伤正气；练功量过小，不足以激发和调动人体正气，难以达到练功目的。对于初学者而言，可首先选择一种姿势练习，时间从20分钟开始，逐步增加到40分钟，再加到60分钟为止，每天练1~2次。

Exercise intensity also varies from person to person. People with chronic illnesses need to pay extra attention to their exercise intensity. Under-exertion cannot active and regulate healthy qi; while overexertion may damage healthy qi. Beginners can start with one posture and practice once or twice a day. At first, you can practice 20 minutes. Gradually, you can increase the exercise time to 40, then 60 minutes.

身体强壮的人可以多采用站式或行式，身体较为虚弱可多采用坐式或卧式以节省体力。在行、站、坐、卧四种姿势中，行式消耗体力最大，体内气血运行最旺盛，但放松较难，尤其是初学者容易开小差；站式消耗体力较小，体内气血运行较快，较容易放松；坐式消耗体力较少，体内气血运行较慢，最容易放松；卧式消耗体力较小，体内气血运行最慢，没有较容易放松，但初学者容易昏沉。

As for body postures, standing or walking is advisable for those with a strong body; and sitting or lying is better for those who are weak. Walking consumes maximal physical strengthen and allows optimal circulation of qi and blood; however, it's very difficult to relax, especially for beginners. Standing consumes less physical strength, allows faster circulation of qi and blood and can easily relax your body and mind. Sitting consumes less physical strength, results in slower circulation of qi and blood and can relax your body and mind very easily. Lying consumes little physical strength, results in slowest circulation of qi and blood and can easily relax your body and mind; however, beginners may feel drowsy.

早上练功可以多练拍打放松法、振颤放松法等动功,有利于气血通畅;晚上睡前,可以多练松通法、三线放松法、分段放松法、局部放松法、整体放松法和倒行放松法等偏于静功的功法,有利于入睡。

It's advisable to practice dynamic exercises such as tapping or shaking/trembling relaxation methods in the morning to circulate qi and blood. Before sleep at night, it's better to practice static exercises such as Relaxing and Unblocking Method, Three-line Relaxation Method, Segmental Relaxation Method, Local Relaxation Method, Whole Body Relaxation Method and Reversed Relaxation Method.

在办公室等公共场合或遇到雷雨天气习练放松功时,不宜入静太深,以免受到干扰,造成惊功现象。在家中,或安全可靠的环境中,可以加深入静程度,取得更好的效果。

When you practice *Fang Song Gong* at home or in a safe

environment, it's advisable to enter deep tranquility for better effect. However, when you practice in public places (e.g. office) or on bad weather days (e.g. thunderstorm), please be sure not to be taken by surprise from sudden interference.

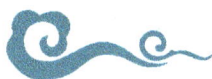

放 松 功　•　*Fang Song Gong* (Relaxation Exercise)

Characteristics and Essential Principles

特色与要领

放松功是所有气功的基础功法

Fang Song Gong serves as the foundation for qigong exercise.

气功功法，不论门派，不外三调，即"调身、调息、调心"。气功锻炼的过程就是不断地对身形、呼吸、意念加以调整，最后达到"三调合一"状态的过程。不论何种功法，在练功前都要先正身、调息、收心，做到身体中正安舒，呼吸均匀柔和，排除杂念，内心平静。在这一过程中，不论身体的"中正安舒""轻灵圆活"，呼吸的"深、长、柔、细"，还是心理的"意守丹田""孤灯寂照"，都是以放松为基础的。

All qigong exercises require three regulations — regulating the body, breathing and mind. These three regulations run through the whole process of qigong practice. Eventually, you can achieve the 'unity of three regulations'. Prior to qigong practice, it's essential to keep the body upright and comfortable, regulate breathing and remove distracting thoughts and concentrate the mind. During this process, relaxation is the precondition for 'upright, comfortable and agile' body, 'deep, long, soft and fine' breathing as well as 'mental consciousness on Dantian' or 'a lonely lamp in quiet stillness'.

在许多门派深入修炼的过程中，也一直伴随着放松功的操作。道家的代表功法周天功，在修炼过程中，只有在身、心放松之后，人体气血运行才会汇聚于丹田。如果肌肉紧张，姿势僵硬,呼吸急促、心烦意乱,真气是难以汇聚在丹田的。在河车搬运的过程中,呼吸的放松是基础,只有在放松的过程中调匀呼吸,才能推动真气的运行。

Fang Song Gong is practiced in deep cultivation of many qigong schools. For example, only with body-mind relaxation, can Daoist Zhou Tian Gong (microcosmic and macrocosmic orbit exercises) allow free flow of qi and blood to Dantian. It's unlikely for genuine qi to gather at Dantian if you have muscular tension, stiff body posture, rapid breathing and restlessness.

佛家的代表功法六妙法门与四禅八定也都是从放松开始的。四禅八定从调心入手,是身心放松,排除杂念之后,才能一步一步地提升功力,如果身体僵硬,杂念丛生,精神紧张,入静的深度是难以提高的。六妙法门从调息入手,身体放松、中正安舒,呼吸才能顺畅,才能逐渐进入"深、长、柔、细"的状态。相反,如果呼吸急促、粗重,是难以深入修炼的。

Relaxation of breathing is the foundation for smooth circulation of qi.The Six Entrances of Enlightenment (Liu Miao Fa Men) in Zen meditation starts from breathing regulation. 'Deep, long, soft and fine' breathing depends on an upright, relaxed and comfortable body. The Four Dhyanas and Eight Samadhis (Si Chan Ba Ding) in Buddhism starts from mind regulation. You cannot enter deep tranquility with body stiffness, distracting thoughts and mental stress.

放松功对于动功也一样重要。不论八段锦、五禽戏,还是其他功法,都是从调身入手,只有身形端正,体内气机才能顺畅,动作才能舒展大方。也只有放松之后,才能进入练功的意境,如五禽戏,要求神似,就是不仅要模仿五种动物的外形,还要模仿五种动物的神态，只有心理放松放下自己原有的心理状态，才能真正地模仿动物的心理状态，才能做到神似。

Fang Song Gong is equally important for dynamic exercises. *Ba Duan Jin, Wu Qin Xi* and other physical exercises all start from body regulation, because an upright relaxed body allows free flow of qi inside the body and subsequently, smooth body movements. Only with relaxation, can you reach the qigong realm. Take *Wu Qin Xi* (Five Animal Frolics) for example, you need to mimic both the appearance and expression of five animals. Only by mental relaxation, can you really imitate the lifelike state of those animals.

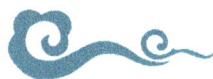

放 松 功　•　*Fang Song Gong* (Relaxation Exercise)

Movements of *Fang Song Gong*

功
法
操
作

基 础 操 作

Basic Movements

放松功的锻炼包括三个方面：身体、呼吸和意念。专业术语分别称为"调身""调息""调心"。调身的内容会告诉我们如何摆放姿势，应该做哪些动作，怎么才能做好这些动作；调息的内容会告诉我们练功时该如何调节、控制自己的呼吸；调心的内容会告诉我们如何控制自己的心理活动。"三调"包括了我们对自身控制的全部内容。"三调"在不同气功功法中的重要性是有差别的，松通法、三线放松法、分段放松法、局部放松法、整体放松法和倒行放松法等静功偏重于调心；振颤放松法、拍打放松法偏重于调身。

Fang Song Gong exercise involves the body, breathing and mental consciousness. In qigong practice, these three aspects are termed as three regulations—regulating the body, breathing and mind. Regulating the body is about the correct body posture and specific body movements; regulating the breathing is about the proper way to control your breathing; and regulating the mind is about the appropriate way to control your mental activities. These three regulations play different roles in different qigong practice. For example, regulating the mind is more stressed in Relaxing and Unblocking Relaxation, Three-Line Relaxation Method, Segmental Relaxtion Method, Local Relaxation Method, Whole Body Relaxation Method and Reversed Relaxation method, whereas regulating the body is more stressed in Trembling and Tapping Relaxation Methods.

调身
Regulating the body

练习放松功的时候有多种姿势可供选择，可以站着练，可以坐着练，可以躺着练，也可以边走边练。我们分别叫做"站式""坐式""卧式""行式"。

Fang Song Gong can be practiced in various postures—standing, sitting, lying or walking.

1. 站式
1. Standing posture

两腿分开，自然站立，以舒适为度；两脚平行，与肩同宽，双膝微曲，膝盖不超出足尖，臀部向下坐，感觉自己好像是坐在凳子上，腰部伸展，不要挺肚子，上身正直，含胸拔背，头颈部正直。轻闭双目，口微闭。两臂自然下垂，松肩垂肘，双手可以自然垂于体侧（站式图1），也可合抱丹田（站式图2），也可以放在身体前面，掌心向内，像抱了一个球一样。

Separate the legs to stand naturally and comfortably. Parallel the feet to shoulder-width apart, slightly bend the knees but do not let the knees go past your toes. Lower down your buttocks to feel like sitting on a stool. Stretch the waist, tuck in the belly and keep the upper body upright. Keep the chest in, pull up the back and keep the head and neck upright. Close your eyes and mouth slightly. Drop your arms and elbows, relax your shoulders and place your hands on front or both sides of the body. Make the palms inward as if holding an inflated balloon. Alternatively, overlap your hands or place your hands on Dantian.(See standing posture 1 and 2)

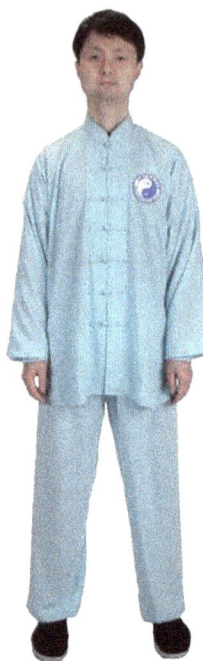

站式图1　Standing posture 1

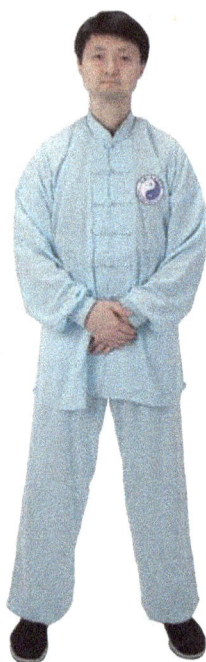

站式图2　Standing posture 2

2. 坐式

2. Sitting posture

　　平坐式：臀部坐在凳子或椅子的外三分之一，不要满坐，凳子或椅子的高度与小腿长度相当，两脚平行分开约与肩同宽，不要八字形，膝关节呈90°，大腿与地面平行，与上身呈90°。腰要直，头要正，下颌微收，舒胸拔背，颈部松直，两眼轻闭，口自然闭合，上下牙齿若接若离，两臂自然下垂，松肩垂肘，双手掌心向下，自然放于大腿上（坐式图1），或平放在小腹部，两肘自然弯曲，使两腋分开，不要夹紧。

　　Flat sitting: Sit on lateral 1/3 of the stool/chair and make the height of the stool/chair match with the length of your lower legs.Separate and parallel the feet to shoulder-width apart and bend the knees to 90°. Be sure your thighs are parallel to the floor and create a 90° angle between your thighs and the upper body. Pull up the waist and back, keep the head upright, slightly tuck in the chin and relax the chest and neck. Close the eyes and mouth and make the upper teeth slightly touch the lower teeth. Drop the arms and elbows and relax the shoulders. Make the palms downward and place the hands on the thighs. Alternatively, place the hands on the lower abdomen, flex the elbows and relax the armpits. (See sitting posture 1)

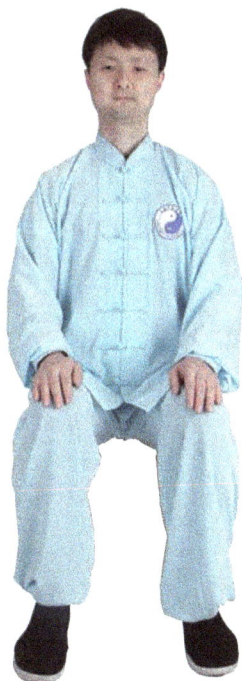

坐式图1　Sitting posture 1

　　靠坐式：坐在床上，背部垫起约45°，头放正，颈部松直，口眼轻闭，四肢自然伸展，两腿可根据个人习惯自然分开或并拢，脚尖自然分向外侧，两臂自然放于体侧，双手掌心向内，或双手重叠放于丹田处。

Backward-leaning sitting: Sit on the bed at approximately 45° with cushion behind the back, keep the head upright and relax the neck. Close the eyes and mouth and stretch the four limbs. Separate the legs or place the legs together, with toes pointing outward. Drop the arms to both sides of the body, make the palms inward or place the overlapped hands on Dantian .

盘坐式：上身同平坐式，两腿相叠。双手掌心向下，自然放于膝关节（坐式图2），或双手相叠放于丹田处。

Sitting with crossed legs: The position of the upper body is same as flat sitting. Cross the legs, make the palms downward and place the hands on knee joints or place the overlapped hands on Dantian. (See sitting posture 2)

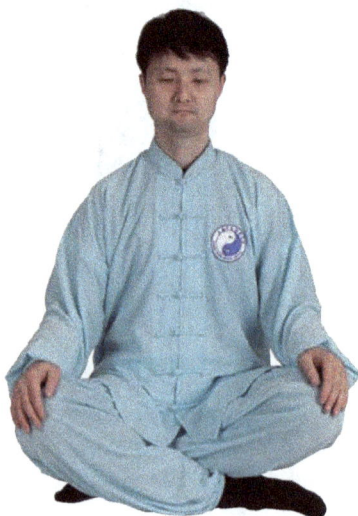

坐式图2　Sitting posture 2

3. 卧式

3. Lying posture

　　躺在床上也有两种姿势，仰卧式与侧卧式。仰卧式时，平躺在床上，面朝上，头正直，口眼轻闭，四肢自然伸展，两腿可根据个人习惯自然分开或并拢，脚尖自然分向外侧，两臂自然向下伸展，双手掌心向内，放于体侧（卧式图1），或双手重叠放于丹田处。

Supine lying: Lie on your back (face up), keep the head upright and close your eyes and mouth. Stretch your limbs and either separate the legs or place them together, with toes pointing outward. Drop the arms, with the palms inward. Place the hands on both sides of the body or place the overlapped hands on Dantian. (See lying posture 1)

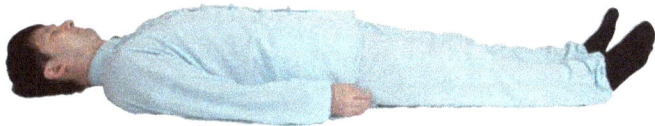

卧式图1　Lying posture 1

　　侧卧位时，侧卧于床，头略向胸部收，双目轻合，两腿叠放，膝部自然弯曲，上方的腿弯曲度数较大，上方的手心向下，放于髋部，下方手臂屈肘，手心向上，放于耳前。左侧卧、右侧卧皆可，但人体心脏在左边，左侧卧位时心脏在下面，容易受压，所以一般以右侧卧为多（卧式图2）。

Side lying: Lie on either side, slightly tilt your head to the chest and close your eyes. Overlap your legs and bend your knees (a larger curvature of the leg on top). Make the palm of the hand on top downward and place on the hip. Flex the arm and elbow of the hand at bottom and place in front of the ear. Since the heart is located in the left side, it's generally to lie on the right side . (See lying posture 2)

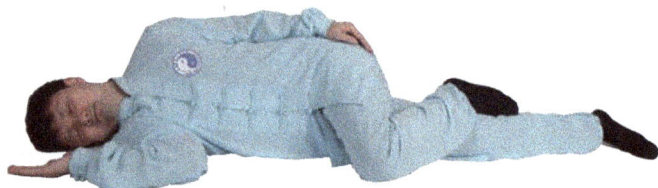

卧式图2　Lying posture 2

4. 行式
4. Walking posture

头正直,双目轻合,目视前方,颈部松直,沉肩,含胸,腰部松直,含胸拔背,两臂自然前后摆动,两腿向前迈步是要放松,步子不要迈得太大,保持身体正直,以缓慢自然的步伐行走。行式因为运动幅度较大,放松有一定难度,初学者不易掌握,随着练功的深入,可逐渐领会。

Keep the head and body upright, slightly close your eyes and look straight ahead. Relax the neck, shoulders and waist, keep the chest in and pull up the back. Swing your arms back and forth and step forward. Be sure your steps are not too big, keep the body upright and walk slowly and comfortably.

这里介绍的姿势比较多,归结起来,调身的要点是全身放松,这些要求都是身体放松过程中逐渐达到的,开始做不到也没有关系,以身体中正,放松为好,随着练功时间的延长,放松程度的加深,身体的姿势就会逐渐调整过来。

In summary, it's essential to keep the body upright and gradually relax the body. It may take some time to adjust the body posture.

调息
Regulating the breathing

1. 呼吸的形式
1.Breathing patterns

自然呼吸：接近我们平时生活中安静状态下的呼吸，练功时略微关注一下呼气，这时的呼吸比我们平时的呼吸略慢，一般来说，一分钟10次左右，是一种略带意念的胸式呼吸。胸式呼吸的特点是呼吸时可见胸部起伏。

Natural breathing: is similar to respiration during rest except for a little more focus on exhalation. Generally it's slower (approximately 10 times per minute) than your usual breathing. Actually it's mental consciousness-involved chest breathing characterized by an upward and outward movement of the chest.

腹式呼吸：腹式呼吸是在自然呼吸的基础上，经过长期锻炼，逐渐形成的一种呼吸形式，主要特点是呼吸时腹部起伏。根据起伏的方式又可细分为顺腹式呼吸与逆腹式呼吸。吸气时如果腹部是隆起的，呼气时腹部是收回的，我们就叫顺腹式呼吸。吸气时如果腹部是收回的，呼气时腹部是隆起的，我们就叫逆腹式呼吸。

Abdominal breathing: is done by contracting the diaphragm on the basis of natural breathing. It's characterized by an outward movement of the abdominal wall. Abdominal breathing can be further subdivided into normal abdominal breathing and reverse abdominal breathing by the outward movement model of the abdominal wall. As for normal abdominal breathing, the abdomen relaxes outward during inhalation and contracts inward during exhalation. As for reverse abdominal breathing, the abdomen contracts inward during inhalation and relaxes outward during exhalation.

发声呼吸：呼气的同时配合发音。放松功里常用的发声呼吸是在呼气时默念"松"。放松功里练功初期也用到发声呼吸，在呼气时默念"松"。随着放松、入静程度的加深，逐渐转为无声呼吸，那是没有了声音，只剩下口型，最后连口型也不做了，只有放松的感觉。

Breathing with sound: refers to aspiration of sound during exhalation. During *Fang Song Gong* exercise, the sound of 'Song' is often aspirated during exhalation.Beginners of *Fang Song gong* also use this breathing with sound and silent aspiration of 'Song'. Over time, along with relaxation and meditation, the breathing has no sound, just the mouth shape. Then even the mouth shape is not necessary, only a feeling of relaxation is felt.

2. 呼吸的境界
2.Breathing realm

古人把呼吸状态描述为四种情况：有声为风，无音为气，出入为息，气出不尽为喘也。具体为：云何为风相？坐时则鼻中息出入觉有声，是风相也。云何为喘相？坐时息虽无声，而出入结滞不通，是喘相也。云何为气相？坐时息虽无声，亦不结滞，而出入不细，是气相也。云何为息相？不声、不结、不粗，出入绵绵,若存若亡,资神安稳,情抱悦豫,此是息相也。

According to ancient Chinese people, there are four breathing states: Wind phase, gasp phase, qi phase and quiescent phase. More specifically, wind phase refers to raspy and noisy breathing through the nose; gasp phase refers to restricted or choppy breathing; qi phase refers to rough breathing and quiescent phase refers to fine and deep breathing.

呼吸气息操作的风相、喘相、气相和息相在练功中各有所用,未必有高下之分。例如,气相是人们自然呼吸时的气息出入之相,其特点是出入无声,但呼与吸之间的转折分明且有少许停顿;风相是需要加大呼吸气息量时而形成的气息出入特征,此时呼吸气息的出或入均带出如风吹过隙之声,故以风名之;喘相在练功中的运用是指有意操作的张口抬肩、气息出入粗犷有力的呼吸气息之相,例如,某些武术气功中发力之前的呼吸。

These four phases play different roles in breathing exercise. For example, qi phase often occurs in natural breathing and is characterized by noiseless inhalation and exhalation, distinct transition and a short pause between inhalation and exhalation; wind phase is characterized by increased respiration rate and noisy (like wind) inhalation and exhalation; gasp phase is characterized by fast breathing with intentional open mouth and raised shoulders, like breathing before exerting force in qigong martial arts.

出入气息的息相用现代语言来描述就是深、长、柔、细,微煦而绵绵不绝的呼吸。这里绵绵不绝的意思是吸气与呼气之间的转折没有痕迹,如同高手拉提琴换弓时琴音不间断一样。这个转折如果有痕迹,呼和吸之间就必然会有间断,气息就不可能绵绵不绝了。古人检测这种形态的气息出入时,将一根羽毛放在鼻孔前,以"鸿毛可以不动"为准。按现代研究,已知平

常人每分钟呼吸是 16~20 次，而练静功时可以减到每分钟10
次一下，甚至数分钟 1 次，此时的呼吸次数减少但并不闭气，即
每次呼吸之间没有停顿，仅是呼和吸的时间均已大大延长。练
放松功所要求的呼吸气息形态是最后一种，即息相，前三种一
般应避免出现。因为"守风则散，守喘则结，守气则劳，守息则
定"。只有"出入绵绵，若存若亡"的息相，才有益于进入高层
次气功境界。

The quiescent phase can be described as deep, long, soft, fine and uninterrupted in modern language. The 'uninterrupted' here means there is no noticeable transition between inhalation and exhalation, like uninterrupted melodic lines in a skillful violin player. In other words, there is no pause between inhalation and exhalation. Ancient people tested this by a little piece of feather remaining still in front of the nostrils. We now know that normally average people breathe 16-20 times per minute. However, during static exercise (meditation), the frequency can be decreased to 1-2 times per minute or once in several minutes. There is no breath holding, i.e., there is no pause between inhalation and exhalation, but greatly lengthened inhalation and exhalation time. As for *Fang Song Gong* practice, it's advisable to avoid the first three phases but use the last phase (quiescent), because wind phase causes mental distraction, gasp phase causes mental stagnation, qi phase causes mental fatigue and quiescent phase leads to mental tranquility.

在此调息操作过程中，要以"勿忘勿助"为原则，既要主动
去调整呼吸，使其向深、长、柔、细、绵绵不绝的方向变化，又不可
故意憋气，勉强去做，须用意不用力。练功过程中出现的胸闷、
头晕、劳累等不适，多与呼吸气息的操作不当有关。待调息有了
一定基础之后，气息的控制过程就有可能由有意识变为下意识。
此时意识对呼吸已并不专门予以注意，只是跟随即可。在放松

功习练过程中运用的是息相，并注重呼气。

It's important to follow the principle of 'do not forget about it but do not try to help it along' in breathing regulation. On one hand, you need actively regulate your breathing to allow it to become deep, long, soft, fine and uninterrupted. On the other hand, do not hold your breath and force yourself to do it (but use your mental intent). Discomforts such as chest tightness, dizziness and exhaustion during qigong practice are often associated with inappropriate breathing exercise. Over time, you may not need to place special attention to breathing any more, but just follow it subconsciously.

调心
Regulating the mind

调心是放松功的核心，也是比较难的地方。放松功常用的调心方法有两种，一种是意守，另一种是观想。

This is the core and difficult part of *Fang Song Gong*. There are two methods to regulate the mind — one is mental concentration and the other is visualization.

1. 意守
1. Mental consciousness

意守就是把意识"轻轻地放在某处"。意守的对象可以是一个部位，也可以是一种感觉。练放松功时常常意守的部位有"丹田、命门、肚脐"，常常意守的是放松后的感觉。具体操作分两步，先把意念从外面收回来，再把意念集中在意守的部位，做到意内守、目内视、耳内听。这里的"内听、内视"指的是意念集中时的感受。需要强调的是"意守"是把意识轻轻地放在丹田，不要太用力。

Mental consciousness means to place your mental focus somewhere naturally. The object of mental consciousness can be a specific body part or a special feeling. Body parts for mental consciousness during qigong practice include Dantian, Mingmen or umbilicus. The special feeling for mental consciousness often occurs after relaxation. There are two steps to concentrate your mind. First, cleanse distracting thoughts and concentrate. Second, focus the mental consciousness on specific body parts. It's required to achieve inner tranquility, inner visualization and listening with the heart. 'Inner visualization' and 'listening with the heart' are feelings upon mental consciousness. It's worth noting that when we say placing your mental consciousness on Dantian, just do it naturally and do not force yourself or you will only generate a new form of tension.

意守不同部位的区别在于不同的穴位本身具有的不同生理效应。根据阴阳理论，阴虚阳亢者宜多练静功，意守涌泉；阴盛阳衰者，宜多练动功，意守命门。

Placing mental consciousness on different points may produce different physiological effects. According to yin-yang theory, those with hyperactivity of yang due to yin deficiency should practice more static exercises and place their mental consciousness on Yongquan (KI 1)[1]; those with yang deficiency should practice more dynamic exercise and place their mental

1. An acupuncture point located on the sole, in the depression appearing on the anterior part of the sole when the foot is in the plantar flexion, approximately at the junction of the anterior third and posterior two thirds of the line connecting the base of the 2nd and 3rd toes and the heel.

consciousness on Mingmen.

丹田：肚脐下3寸（肚脐到耻骨联合共5寸），相当于任脉关元穴的位置。在实际练功时，人们是无法将意念仅仅守在一个点上，只能意守在以穴位为中心的一个范围。古人练气功时对丹田极为重视，道家认为丹田是储藏精气神的地方，是运行小周天的起点。意守丹田可以激发体内的能量物质，充实下元，具有防止早衰，健身延年的作用。

Dantian is located at 3 cun (proportional measurement, 5 cun from the umbilicus to symphysis pubis) below the umbilicus, at the same location of Guanyuan (Ren 4). However, during qigong practice, rather than a small point, people often place their mental consciousness on a small area centered on that point. Ancient people believed Dantian is extremely important. From Daoist perspective, Dantian stores essence, qi and spirit and is therefore the origin of microcosmic orbit. Placing mental consciousness on Dantian can activate internal energy, benefit the kidney, prevent premature aging and achieve longevity.

肚脐：在脐窝正中，是任脉上重要的穴位。是胎儿出生前从母体获取营养的通道，在胚胎发育过程中为腹壁直接相连，内联十二经脉、五脏六腑、四肢百骸、五宫、皮肉筋，因而历来被医家视为治病要穴。

Umbilicus is located at the center of navel recess. It is also an important point along the Ren meridian. As a conduit between the developing embryo or fetus and the placenta, umbilicus is directly associated with the abdominal walls during prenatal development. Since it's connected with twelve regular meridians, five-zang organs, four limbs, five sense organs, skin, muscles and sinews, it's been highly valued by physicians in different generations as a key point for disease treatment.

命门：命门穴位于督脉，腰椎二三棘突间。中医学认为命门蕴藏先天之气，集中体现肾的功能，故对五脏六腑的功能发挥着决定性的作用。在男子能藏生殖之精，在女子则紧密联系着胞宫，对两性生殖功能有重要影响。命门内含有真阳(真火)、真阴(真水)，五脏六腑以及整个人体的生命活动都由它激发和主持。但是，也有人持命门只含真火而不含真水的见解。近代的观点，多倾向于命门主要是藏"真火"，因而称之为"命门火"或"命火"。由于肾脏是"先天之本""水火之宅"，所以不论从上述哪种观点来看，命门的功能都与肾脏有十分密切的关系。

Mingmen (DU 4), literally means vital gate (or gate of life), is located in the depression below the spinous process of the 2nd lumbar vertebra. According to Chinese medicine, Mingmen stores congenital qi, manifests functions of the kidney and thus plays a decisive role in regulating functions of the five-zang and six-fu organs. For men, it stores the reproductive essence. For women, it is closely associated with the uterus. What's more, Mingmen contains genuine yang (fire) and genuine yin (water) and therefore activates and dominates all vital activities. However, some people believe Mingmen only contains genuine fire. Contemporary scholars tend to believe Mingmen mainly stores genuine fire, known as 'vital fire' or 'fire of the vital gate'. Anyway, Mingmen is closely associated with the kidney because kidney is considered as the 'congenital root' and 'house of genuine water and fire'.

意守丹田或肚脐重在培补元气。意守命门重在强腰补肾。也可以选择丹田、肚脐、命门中的两个或三个部位相继意守。

Placing mental consciousness on Dantian or umbilicus

helps to cultivate yuan-primordial qi, whereas placing mental consciousness on Mingmen helps to benefit the kidney and strengthen the waist. You can place your mental consciousness on two of them or three in succession.

意守时，不要用力守，只要把意念轻轻地放在那里就好，要做到"似守非守"。如果一时找不到丹田等部位的感觉，不要着急，只需静静地等待，丹田处的感觉就会自然出现。

Tips Do not force yourself into mental concentration. Just place your mental consciousness there naturally. The ideal state is to keep the mental consciousness to 'focus there but not there'. In case you cannot obtain the feeling of Dantian, just be patient and wait.

---

2. 观想
2.Inner visualization

观想又称存想，想象特定的景物，或亲身经历的身心状态。在放松功中，可以观想有水流从身体中流过，或者身体像海绵一样等。意守和观想的区别在于意守对象多为现实存在事物，而观想对象或内容大多是练功者想象出来的，在现实中并不存在或当下并不存在。例如，观想一轮明月当空，而练功时很可能是阴天，根本看不到月亮。

Visualization, also known as contemplation, means to imagine specific scenes or experiencing specific body-mind state. During *Fang Song Gong* practice, you can visualize water flowing through the body or feeling like a sponge. Mental consciousness is different from inner visualization in that it focuses on real objects instead of imagination. For example, when practicing *Fang Song Gong* in cloudy days, you can still visualize a bright moon shining in the sky.

观想的内容不同产生的效果也不同,例如,观想月亮、流水,会使人平静;观想太阳、火焰,会让人活跃甚至感到温暖。观想静止的东西更有利于入静,例如,在练功前,观想平静的水面有助于快速安静下来,进入练功状态;观想运动的物体有利于气血流动,例如在做整体放松功时,观想水流从头顶向下流过,或电波从丹田向外扩散,都有利于放松部位逐渐扩大。

Different things in visualization may produce different effects. For example, visualization of moon and running water can make you calm down; visualization of sun and flame can make you active and warm. Visualization of static things can help you into tranquility, for example, visualization of motionless water can help you calm down and enter a qigong state; visualization of dynamic things can help with the circulation of qi and blood, for example, when practicing whole body relaxation, visualization of water running down from top of the head or electric wave spreading from Dantian can help to enlarge the relaxation area.

具 体 操 作
Individual Movements

放松功包括功前准备、主体功法、功后动作三部分。

Fang Song Gong includes three parts—Preparation, principal movements and movements after conclusion.

功前准备
Warm-up exercise

作好功前准备，可以减少练功中一些杂念，有助于提高练功质量，保持练功的顺利进行。一般在练功前5~10分钟进行。

This can be done 5 to 10 minutes before *Fang Song Gong*. These warm-up activities help to remove distracting thoughts and improve the exercise quality.

（1）先使情绪稳定下来，停止原来的一些活动，包括工作、学习、阅读、思考、文娱活动等。如感到太疲劳或心情烦躁时，可暂不练功。

（1）Discontinue ongoing activities including work, study, reading, thinking and recreation to stabilize emotions. Do not force yourself to practice if you feel tired or upset.

（2）练功场所的光线不要太强，空气要流通，但避免直接吹风。

（2）Make sure the exercise place to have good ventilation, soft light and no direct wind exposure.

（3）周围环境要保持比较安静，一般应避免在练功时有剧烈声响发生。

（3）Keep the exercise place quiet; it's essential to prevent loud sudden noise.

（4）患者局部疼痛或临床症状比较明显而影响练功时，可先采取一些对症措施。

（4）Take some measures to deal with localized pain or discomfort before the practice of *Fang Song Gong*.

（5）安排好练功用的卧床和坐椅，力求合适。床一般以木板床较好。坐椅高低适宜，坐椅太高，脚底下垫物；坐椅太低，垫高坐椅。

（5）Make sure the (wooden) bed and chair (height) for exercise are comfortable.

（6）如有必要，可先排除大小便。

（6）It's better to empty the bladder and bowel before the practice of *Fang Song Gong*.

（7）松开衣领、腰带等束紧在身上的东西。衣着既不要太紧，也不要松散。

（7）Loosen the collar or belt and make the clothes not too

tight or loose.

（8）先做三节保健功：叩齿、搅海咽津、摩腹。

（8）Perform the following three health care exercises: click the teeth, swallow saliva and rub the abdomen.

叩齿：把牙齿上下叩合，先叩大牙3次，再叩前牙3次。可帮助集中注意，有坚齿益精作用。

Click the teeth: click the molar teeth 24 times and front teeth 24 times. This helps to concentrate the mind, strengthen the teeth and benefit essence.

搅海咽津：用舌头在牙齿的外上、外下、里上、里下，依次轻轻搅动各6次。先左后右，不要勉强用力。然后舌尖轻抵上额，注意舌下部位，待唾液增多，鼓漱三下，分3次咽下去。能滋润肠胃，帮助消化，改善口苦口臭。

Swallow saliva: Rotate the tongue towards outer upper, outer lower, inner upper and inner lower directions, 9 times in each direction. First, rotate to left side and then to right side. Do not use force. After this, touch the upper palate with the tongue tip until you get a mouthful of saliva and swallow in one or several gulps. This helps to moisten the stomach and intestines, increase digestion and eliminate a bitter taste and foul breath.

摩腹：两手搓热，然后相叠（一般右手按在左手背上），用掌心在脐的周圈，先顺时针，再逆时针各3圈，以顺时针为例（功前准备图1～图4），要点是用腰的运动带动手的运动。

Rub the abdomen: Twist the hands until they become

warm. Overlap the hands (the right hand on top of the dorsum of the left hand) and use the palm to rub the periumbilical area clockwise, 12 times in each circle (a small, medium and big one). This helps to regulate gastrointestinal functions.(See warm-up exercise 1–4)

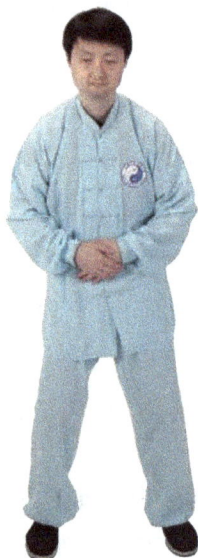

功前准备图1　warm-up exercise 1

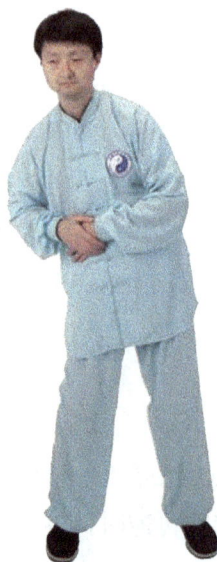

功前准备图2　warm-up exercise 2

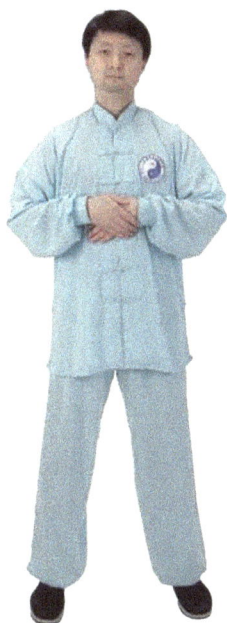

功前准备图 3　warm-up exercise 3

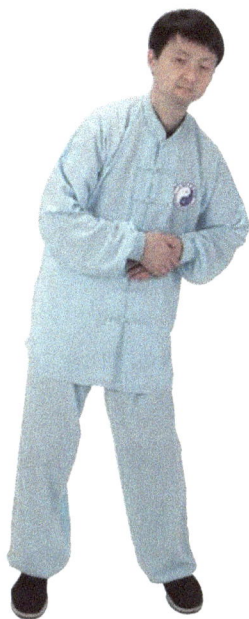

功前准备图 4　warm-up exercise 4

主体功法
Principal Exercise

　　主体功法包括松通法、三线放松法、分段放松法、局部放松法、整体放松法和倒行放松法、振颤放松法和拍打放松法。这些功法具有许多相似之处，例如，松通法、三线放松法、分段放松法、局部放松法、整体放松法可选用的姿势基本相同，站、坐、卧、行都可以练习。这些放松方法都把重点放在了心理调节上，通过不同的心理操作，达到身心放松的目的。振颤放松法和拍打放松法偏于动功，站、坐、行都可以练习。这两种方法对意念的要求不高，重点放在了身体动作的调节上。

Principal exercise of *Fang Song Gong* includes relaxation and unblocking method (*Song Tong Fa*), three-line relaxation method (*San Xian Fang Song Fa*), segmental relaxation method (*Fen Duan Fang Song Fa*), local relaxation method (*Ju Bu Fang*

Song Fa), whole body relaxation method (*Zheng Ti Fang Song Fa*), Reversed Relaxation Method (*Dao Xing Fang Song Fa*), Shaking/Trembling Relaxation Method (*Zhen Chan Fang Song Fa*) and Tapping Relaxation Method (*Pai Da Fang Song Fa*). These methods (for example, relaxing and unblocking method, three-line relaxation method, segmental relaxation method and whole body relaxation method) share same postures in standing, sitting, lying and walking. They focus on mental regulation and body-mind relaxation. Shaking/trembling and tapping relaxation methods are performed in standing, sitting or walking. They focus more on body movements instead of mental concentration.

松通法
Relaxing and Unblocking Method

松通法是有意识地将身体从上到下进行放松，要求目内视、意内想、耳内听、结合默念"松——"字或体会放松的感觉，从而使身心都得到放松的方法。

This method relaxes the body intentionally from top to bottom. It requires inner visualization, inner meditation, inner listening and silent reading of the sound 'song' or experiencing the feeling of relaxation.

习练松通法共有3个步骤（或称三节），第一步顺序放松，第二步意守丹田，第三步玉液还丹。练功的姿势较为多样，站、坐、卧、行皆可，重点在于调心，就是对心理活动的控制。习练时每个部位反复操作3~5次，完整习练一遍松通法的时间一般不少于10分钟。

There are three steps in this method: first, to relax by the sequence; second, focus mental consciousness on Dantian; and third, swallow saliva to Dantian. These steps emphasize mental regulation and can be done in standing, sitting, lying or walking. Repeat 3-5 times on each body part and it often takes at least 10 minutes to finish the whole set.

第一步　全身放松

Step # 1　Relax the whole body

采用站、坐、卧、行的任意一种（要领及图见"基本操作"）。

Posture: Standing, sitting, lying or walking (please refer to 'Basic Movements' for essential principles).

用自然呼吸或腹式呼吸。一般情况下，呼气的时间比吸气的时间略长，在呼气时默念"松——"字。

Breathing: Natural or abdominal breathing. Generally, exhalation is slightly longer than inhalation. Aspirate the sound 'Song' silently during exhalation.

随着引导词从上到下，按序一个部位接着一个部位进行放松。放松的顺序是：头→颈→肩→上臂→肘关节→前臂→腕关节→手→胸背→腰腹→髋关节→大腿→膝关节→小腿→踝关节→脚。

Follow the guide words to relax the body by the sequence of: head → neck → shoulders → upper arms → elbow joints → forearms → wrist joints → hands → chest and back → waist and abdomen → hip joints → thighs → knee joints→ lower legs → ankle joints → feet.

练功时要注意意念、呼吸的协调一致。呼气时默念"松——"字，意念按顺序一个部位连着一个部位往下移。意念操作有两种，第一种是用心听自己念出的"松——"字；第二种是把意识放在放松的感觉上，默念"松——"时，体会那个部位放松的感觉。

Tips Coordinate mental consciousness and breathing. Aspirate the sound 'Song' during exhalation. Move your mental consciousness by the sequence. There are two methods to guide your mental consciousness: one is to listen to the sound of 'Song' with your heart and the other is to experience the feeling of relaxation in that specific body part.

第二步　意守丹田

Step # 2　Focus mental consciousness on Dantian

身体保持上一步的姿势不变。站式、坐式、仰卧式的双手相叠，放在丹田处。一般男性左手在内，女性右手在内，两手要轻轻地放在丹田处，不要用力按。侧卧式的姿势，以右侧卧位为例，左手轻轻放于下丹田处，右手置于耳前即可。左侧卧位与之相反。行式的操作时两臂可自然轻松摆动，也可以双手相叠，放在丹田处。也可以意守肚脐或命门。

Keep the same posture as the first step. As for standing, sitting or supine-lying postures, place the overlapped hands on Dantian gently and do not use pressure. Generally, men place the left hand beneath the right hand and women place the right hand beneath the left hand. As for side-lying posture, for example the right side-lying posture, place the left hand gently on the lower Dantian and the right hand in front of the ear. Do the opposite for left side-lying posture. As for walking, naturally swing the arms or place the overlapped hands on Dantian.

Alternatively, focus mental consciousness on the umbilicus or Mingmen (literally means gate of life and located on the posterior median line, in the depression below the spinous process of the 2nd lumbar vertebra).

呼吸仍采用自然呼吸或腹式呼吸。这时不用再念"松"字了，只要保持深、长、柔、细的呼吸就可以了。

Breath: Natural or abdominal breathing. Just keep deep, long, soft and fine breathing and no need to aspirate the sound of 'Song'.

第三步　玉液还丹
Step # 3　Swallow saliva to Dantian

保持上一步的姿势不变。把口中的唾液分3次咽下。吞咽时要轻柔，不要用力下咽。保持深、长、柔、细的呼吸。

Keep the same posture as the second step. Swallow the saliva gently (do not use force) in three gulps. Maintain the deep, long, soft and fine breathing.

咽唾液时意想体内真气随着口中唾液下至丹田。经过前面的放松、意守，练功者口中唾液分泌会大量增加，到了收功阶段，口中唾液常常很多，这些唾液在古人看来是十分宝贵的，千万不可吐掉。咽完唾液后，两手相搓，做干洗面，梳头，缓慢转动颈部，肩部，活动腰部等动作收功。

When swallowing the saliva, use your mind to guide the saliva down to Dantian. Through the previous relaxation and mental focus, you often have increased saliva in your mouth.

Swallow the saliva, twist the hands to wash your face, comb your hair and slowly turn your neck, shoulder and waist to conclude.

松通法引导词：

Guide words for relaxing and unblocking method:

现在开始练功了，停止工作，请安静下来，在正式练功前，先调整好姿势——调匀呼吸——保持平静的心态——

Before the practice of relaxing and unblocking method, let's adjust our posture, breath naturally and keep a peaceful mind.

在放松的过程中，你要做的只是跟随口令，轻轻地体会放松的感觉。

What we need to do is to follow the word of command and experience the feeling of relaxation.

现在开始练功：先把意念集中在头部，头部放松 ——
松——松——→颈部放松——松——松——→肩部放松——
松——松——→上臂放松——松——松——→肘部放松——
松——松——→前臂放松——松——松——→手腕部放松——
松——松——→手部放松——松——松——→胸背放松——
松——松——→腰腹放松——松——松——→臀部放松——
松——松——→大腿放松——松——松——→膝关节放松——
松——松——→小腿放松——松——松——→脚踝放松——
松——松——→脚部放松——松——松——

Now let's start. Relax the head—Song—Song → relax

the neck — Song—Song → relax the shoulders — Song—Song → relax the upper arms — Song—Song → relax the elbow joints — Song — Song → relax the forearms — Song — Song → relax the wrist joints — Song — Song → relax the hands — Song — Song → relax the chest and back — Song — Song → relax the waist and abdomen — Song — Song → relax the buttocks — Song — Song → relax the thighs — Song — Song → relax the knee joints — Song — Song → relax the lower legs — Song — Song → relax the ankle joints — Song — Song → relax the feet — Song — Song.

身体已经完全放松了, 现在把意识轻轻地放到丹田——意守丹田——做3次深呼吸——

Now let's place our mental focus on Dantian, concentrate on Dantian and take 3 times of deep breathing.

现在把口中唾液分3次咽下, 第一次——第二次——第三次——

Now let's swallow the saliva in three gulps, one — two — three.

现在开始收功: 轻轻地搓动两手——从练功状态慢慢地恢复到生活状态——

Now let's conclude: twist the hands gently and return to a normal state from qigong state.

练功到此结束。

The end.

三线放松法
Three-line Relaxation Method

三线放松法是将身体分部位放松的一种方法，它将人体划分成侧面、前面、后面三条线，每条线又分为9个放松部位和1个止息点，练功时沿此三条线路自上而下依次进行放松。按顺序完成三线各部位的放松与意守，作为一个循环。每次锻炼可练1个循环，也可练2~3个循环。完整练习一遍三线放松法的时间应该不少于10分钟。三线放松法是放松功的基本方法之一。

As a basic relaxation method, this exercise relaxes the body from top to bottom by three lines, namely the lateral line, anterior line and posterior line. Each line is subdivided into nine body parts and an end point. One cycle includes relaxation and mental focus of all body parts along the three lines. Every time one can practice one cycle or 2-3 cycles. It takes at least 10 minutes to finish the whole set.

这一步的姿势可采用站、坐、卧、行的任意一种。侧卧位时，上面的侧线较容易放松，如果要放松下面的一条侧线，最好翻个身，更换一下体位。仰卧位时，后面的一条侧线如果难以放松，可以选择侧卧位放松后面一条线路，等后面一条路放松后，再恢复仰卧位。

Posture: standing, sitting, lying or walking. In side-lying position, it's easier to relax the lateral line on top. To relax the lateral line at the bottom, it's better to roll over the body. To relax the posterior line in a supine-lying position, it's better to change to side-lying position and then return the supine-lying position.

三线放松法可采用自然呼吸或腹式呼吸。吸气时意守一个部位。呼气时默念"松——"。吸气时再意守下一个部位，呼气时默念"松——"。如此循环。

Breathing: Natural or abdominal breathing. Focus mental consciousness on one body part during inhalation. Aspirate the sound of 'Song' during exhalation. Then shift the mental consciousness to next body part during inhalation and aspirate the sound of 'Song' during exhalation.

调心操作可以体会身体各部位放松的感觉。

Mental regulation can help you to experience the feeling of relaxation in different body parts.

三条线路分别为：

The three lines are as follows:

第一条线：头部两侧→颈部两侧→两肩→两上臂→两肘→两前臂→两腕→两手→十个手指。止息点是中冲穴。

Line # 1: both sides of the head → both sides of the neck → shoulders → upper arms → elbows→ forearms → wrists → hands→ ten fingers. End point: Zhongchong (PC 9, located at the tip of the middle finger).

第二条线：面部→颈前→胸部→腹部→两大腿前→两膝→两小腿→两脚→十个脚趾。止息点是隐白穴。

Line # 2: Face → front of the neck → chest → abdomen→ front of the thighs → knees → lower leg → feet → ten toes. End point: Yinbai (SP 1 located at 0.1 cun from the medial corner of the big toenail).

第三条线：后脑部→后颈→背部→腰部→大腿后→两膝窝→小腿后→两足跟→两脚底。止息点是涌泉穴。

Line # 3: Occiput → back of the neck → back → lower back → back of the thighs→ popliteal fossae → back of the lower legs→ heels — soles. End point: Yongquan (KI 1, located on the sole, in the depression appearing on the anterior part of the sole when the foot is in the plantar flexion, approximately at the junction of the anterior third and posterior two thirds of the line connecting the base of the 2nd and 3rd toes and the heel).

三条线上的所有部位全部放松完毕后，轻轻地意守下丹田3~4分钟。

After relaxing all body parts along the three lines, focus the mental consciousness on lower Dantian for 3-4 minutes.

三线放松法引导词：

Guide words for three-line relaxation method:

现在开始练功了，停止工作，请安静下来，在正式练功前，先调整好姿势——调匀呼吸——保持平静的心态——

Before the practice of the three-line relaxation method, let's adjust our posture, breath naturally and keep a peaceful mind.

在放松的过程中，你要做的只是跟随口令，轻轻地体会放松的感觉。

What we need to do is to follow the word of command and experience the feeling of relaxation.

现在开始练功：

Now let's start.

第一条线：身体两边放松——先把意念集中在头部→头部两侧放松——松——松——→颈部两侧放松——松——松——→肩膀放松——松——松——→上臂放松——松——松——→肘部放松——松——松——→前臂放松——松——松——→手腕放松——松——松——→手部放松——松——松——→手指放松——松——松——→中冲穴放松——松——松——。

Line # 1: Relax both sides of the body. Relax both sides of the head — Song — Song → relax both sides of the neck — Song — Song → relax the shoulders — Song — Song → relax the upper arms — Song — Song → relax the elbows — Song — Song → relax the forearms — Song — Song → relax the wrists — Song — Song → relax the hands — Song — Song → relax the fingers — relax Zhongchong (PC 9) — Song — Song.

第二条线：身体前面放松——先把意念集中在头部→面部放松——松——松——→脖子前面放松——松——松——→胸部放松——松——松——→腹部放松——松——松——→两大腿前放松——松——松——→膝关节放松——松——松——→小腿放松——松——松——→两脚放松——松——松——→脚趾放松——松——松——→隐白穴放松——松——松——。

Line # 2: Relax front of the body. Relax the face — Song — Song → relax the front of the neck — Song — Song → relax the chest — Song — Song →relax the abdomen — Song — Song →relax the front of the thighs — Song — Song → relax the knee joints — Song — Song → relax the lower legs — Song — Song → relax the feet — Song — Song → relax the toes — Song — Song →relax Yinbai

(SP 1) — Song — Song.

第三条线：身体后面放松——先把意念集中在头部→头的后部放松——松——松——→脖子后面放松——松——松——→背部放松——松——松——→腰部放松——松——松——→大腿后面放松——松——松——→两个膝窝放松——松——松——→小腿后面放松——松——松——→脚跟放松——松——松——→脚底放松——松——松——→涌泉穴放松——松——松——

Line # 3: Relax back of the body. Relax the occiput — Song — Song →relax the back of the neck — Song — Song → relax the back — Song — Song →relax the waist — Song — Song →relax the back of the thighs — Song — Song →relax the popliteal fossae — Song — Song →relax the back of the lower legs — Song — Song →relax the heels — Song — Song →relax the soles — Song — Song →relax Yongquan (KI 1) — Song — Song.

身体已经完全放松了，把意识轻轻地放到丹田——意守丹田——

Now let's place our mental focus on Dantian, concentrate on Dantian and take 3 times of deep breathing.

现在做3次深呼吸——把口中唾液分3次咽下，第一次——第二次——第三次——

Now let's swallow the saliva in three gulps, one — two — three.

现在开始收功：轻轻地搓动两手，从练功状态慢慢地恢复到生活状态。

Now let's conclude: twist the hands gently and return to a normal state from qigong state.

练功到此结束。

The end.

分段放松法
Segmental Relaxation Method

分段放松法是将身体逐段进行放松，要求目内视、意内想、耳内听、结合默念"松——"字和存想放松部位感觉，从而达到放松的目的方法。习练时每个部位反复操作3~5次，完整练习一遍分段法的时间应该不少于10分钟。

This method relaxes the body by segments. It requires inner visualization, inner meditation, inner listening and silent reading of the sound 'song' or experiencing the feeling of relaxation. Repeat 3-5 times on each segment and it often takes at least 10 minutes to finish the whole set.

分段放松法与松通法较为相似，练功的姿势较为多样，站、坐、卧、行皆可。呼吸多采用自然呼吸或腹式呼吸。习练分段放松法时存想的部位范围较大，一般将身体粗略地分为几段，例如，头→胸→腹→上肢→下肢等。在放松过程中，可以将每一个部位作为一个整体进行放松。例如，放松头部时，就将头部作为一个整体，在默念"松"字时体会头部放松的感觉，不要过分关注某些器官的具体感受。在逐渐放松后，某些感官会变得比较敏感，例如用眼疲劳后，眼部会有酸胀感，吃过辛辣食物后，口腔会比较敏感等，这时轻轻地把意识拉回来，仍以关注整个头部为主。胸、腹也同样以整体观觉为主。

Just like relaxing and unblocking method, segmental relaxation method can be performed in standing, sitting, lying or walking. One can use natural or abdominal breathing. Focus mental consciousness on bigger body area, for example head → chest → abdomen → upper limbs → lower limbs, etc. Use each segment as a whole during relaxation. For example, relax the head as a whole when relaxing the head; in other words, experience the feeling of whole head relaxation when aspirating the sound of 'Song' and do not focus on feeling of specific sense organs. However, some sense organs may become sensitive after relaxation. For example, soreness or distension of the eyes may occur upon eye fatigue; or the mouth became more sensitive after eating hot spicy food. Gently re-focus the mental consciousness on the whole head. Likewise, the chest and abdomen are considered as a unit.

分段放松法分为三步（或称四步），第一步顺序放松，第二步意守丹田或命门，第三步玉液还丹。习练者可以根据自己的喜好或身体状态进行选取。

There are three steps in this method: first, to relax by the sequence; second, focus mental consciousness on Dantian or Mingmen; and third, swallow saliva to Dantian. One can choose different steps according to one's preference or individualized physical condition.

分段放松法引导词：

Guide words for segmental relaxation method:

现在开始练功了，停止工作，请安静下来，在正式练功前，先调整好姿势——调匀呼吸——保持平静的心态——

Before the practice of segmental relaxation method, let's adjust our posture, breath naturally and keep a peaceful mind.

在放松的过程中，你要做的只是跟随口令，轻轻地体会放松的感觉。

What we need to do is to follow the word of command and experience the feeling of relaxation.

现在开始练功：先把意念集中在头部，头部放松——松——松——→胸背部放松——松——松——→腰腹部放松——松——松——→上肢放松——松——松——→下肢放松——松——松——

Now let's start. Relax the head — Song — Song → relax the chest and back — Song — Song → relax the waist and abdomen — Song — Song → relax the upper limbs — Song — Song → relax the lower limbs — Song — Song.

身体已经完全放松了，现在把意识轻轻地放到丹田——意守丹田——

Now let's place our mental focus on Dantian, concentrate on Dantian and take 3 times of deep breathing.

做3次深呼吸——把口中唾液分3次咽下，第一次——第二次——第三次——

Now let's swallow the saliva in three gulps, one — two — three.

现在开始收功：轻轻地搓动两手，从练功状态慢慢地恢复到生活状态。

Now let's conclude: twist the hands gently and return to a normal state from qigong state.

练功到此结束。

The end.

局部放松法
Local Relaxation Method

局部放松法是针对身体某一局部有针对性的放松一种方法。习练时可以选取站、坐、卧、行中的任意一种。呼吸多采用自然呼吸或腹式呼吸。调心操作可以体会放松部位感觉。

This method is oriented at specific body parts and can be performed in standing, sitting, lying or walking.

Breathing: Natural or abdominal breathing.

As for mental regulation, one can experience the feeling of relaxation.

局部放松既包含了身、心两个方面，也蕴含着很多层次。随着练功时间的积累，功夫不断地深入，放松的操作方法、操作内容也会发生相应的变化。

Local relaxation contains multiple levels other than body and mind. Over time, the exercise method and contents change accordingly.

下面以眼部为例讲一下放松时的操作与感受。
Take the eyes as example for the feeling of relaxation.

开始放松眼睛的时候，感觉可能很粗，意识所能关注到的眼睛和眼睛周围，只是模糊的一大片部位，甚至感觉不到眼睛是紧张的，这时我们放松的操作也很粗，只是呼气时默念"松"，别的几乎做不了什么。这时不要心急，只要静下心来，摆正姿势，调匀呼吸，慢慢体会，我们的心就会平静下来，呼吸也会变得缓慢而均匀。逐渐的，我们越来越平静，感觉也越来越细致，这时我们会发现自己的眼部原来是紧张的，或许眼球是干涩的，或许眉头皱得太紧，或许眼睛闭得太紧了，转动起来并不灵活，这时放松的操作也随之细化了。如果是眉头太紧，我们可以舒展几下眉头；如果闭得太紧，我们可以眨几下眼睛，放松眼睑；如果眼睛干涩，可以闭着眼睛，轻轻地上下左右活动一下眼球。不需要很久，随着气血的通畅，我们的眉头就会舒展开来，眼睛也不会闭得太紧，我们的眼睛湿润了，眼球活动起来就会灵活些。这时我们不经意间会发现内心更加平静了，呼吸也更加缓慢均匀了，默念"松"字也更加轻了，身体姿势不正，气血不通畅的人还常伴有身体姿势的调整。如果我们坚持练功，继续放松，我们眼部的感觉就会更加细微，眉头已经松开，我们会感到眉头与前额、鼻子其实是连在一起的，眼放松的感觉会带动周边部位的放松，其实眉头太紧和眼睛闭得太紧也是连在一起的。随着放松的深入，上下眼睑也就不会再闭得那么紧了，而是似开未开，似闭微闭，这时，我们的眼球转动灵活了，眼睛更加湿润了，有的人甚至会流出眼泪来。这时我们的内心会变得更加平静，所有的烦恼都消失了，呼吸也变得更加均匀、柔和，默念"松"字，会变得更轻、更细，甚至自己也只能感觉到，而听不到了。随着练功的深入，会逐渐感到眼球深部，甚至是眼底的放松。随着眼底的放松，眼前也不再那么黑暗，而是有了一种微微发白的感觉，随着练功时间的延长，功夫的深入，放松程度会越来越深，不断进入新的放松境界，还会出现许多新的感觉。

When you start to relax the eyes, you may only have a vague feeling. As a result, you may only sense a vague area when you try to focus your mental consciousness on the eyes and their surrounding area. You cannot even tell your eyes are strained. What you can do is to aspirate the sound of 'Song' silently during exhalation. Just be patient and calm down. Adjust your posture, breath naturally and slowly experience. Over time, you start to calm down and have more delicate feelings. Until then you know your eyes are strained: your eyes may be dry, you may frown (the brows are too tight), or you closed your eyes too hard. By now, you can relax the specific eye area. If the brows are too tight, loosen the brows; if the eyes are closed too hard, blink your eyes to relax the eyelids; and if the eyes are dry, close the eyes and gently move the eyeballs upward, downward, leftward and rightward. It won't take long to loosen the brows, moisten the eyes and move the eyeballs. In addition, you feel more calmed, along with slower and more even breathing and easier aspiration of the sound 'Song'. Those with an inappropriate posture and unsmooth flow of qi and blood may also need to adjust their positions. If you continue relaxing, you can feel your brows are loosened, and actually the brows are connected with the forehead and nose. Relaxation of the eyes can help to relax the surrounding area of the eyes. Actually tight brows are associated with too tight closure of the eyes. If you continue relaxing the eyes, you can feel the eyelids are half closed and half open, your eyes become wet and your eyeballs are movable, some people may even have tears. At the same time, all worries are gone, and you become more and more calmed, along with more gentle, even breathing. The sound of 'Song' becomes so gentle that you cannot hear but can only feel. Gradually, you feel relaxed in the deeper area of the eyes, including the eye ground. Then little by little, you feel somewhat white (instead of darkness) in front of your eyes…. Over time, you can become more and more relaxed and may have other new feelings.

当然，这一切不会一下子产生，而是要静下心来体会，日积月累，随着功夫的深入，每个人都会有自己的体会。这种体会需要静下心来，不能执着，我们要做的是静下心等待放松程度的逐渐深入，放松境界自己的提高，而不是刻意地追求某种感觉，如果用心太过，刻意追求，不仅不利于放松，甚至还会适得其反，加重紧张程度。一般来说人和人之间的感觉和反映是有差别的，所以，练功过程中的体会也千差万别，不尽相同，但感觉越来越细微，越来越放松这个方向是相同的。

It takes a long period of time to have the above-mentioned feelings. You need to be really patient to wait for your experience. Obsessive pursuit of those feelings may lead to the opposite to what you wish. In addition, experience may vary from person to person. However, all share the same direction — more subtle feelings and more relaxation.

眼睛放松法引导词：

Guided words for eye relaxation method:

现在开始练功了，停止工作，请安静下来，在正式练功前，先调整好姿势——调匀呼吸——保持平静的心态——

Before the practice of local relaxation method, let's adjust our posture, breath naturally and keep a peaceful mind.

在放松的过程中，你要做的只是跟随口令，轻轻地体会放松的感觉。

What we need to do is to follow the word of command and experience the feeling of relaxation.

现在开始练功：先把意识集中到眼部，眼睛放松——微闭双眼——松——松——眼睑放松——松——松——眼睛湿润一——眼睛湿润二——眼睛湿润三——眉头松开一——眉头松开二——眉头松开三——面部放松一——面部放松二——面部放松三——眼底放松一——眼底放松二——眼底放松三——整个眼部放松一——整个眼部放松二——整个眼部放松三——

Now let's start. Relax the eyes — slight close the eyes — relax the eyelids — Song — Song → eyes become wet (1) — eyes continue to become wet (2)-eyes further continue to become wet (3) — loosen the brows (1) — continue to loosen the brows (2) — further continue to loosen the brows (3) — relax the face (1) — relax the face (2) — relax the face (3) — relax the eye ground (1) — continue to relax the eye ground (2) — further relax the eye ground (3) — relax the eyes (1) — relax the eyes (2) — relax the eyes (3).

眼睛已经完全放松了，现在把意识轻轻地放到丹田——意守丹田——做3次深呼吸——

Now let's place our mental focus on Dantian, concentrate on Dantian and take 3 times of deep breathing.

现在把口中唾液分3次咽下，第一次——第二次——第三次——

Now let's swallow the saliva in three gulps, one — two —

three.

现在开始收功：轻轻地搓动两手——从练功状态慢慢地恢复到生活状态——

Now let's conclude: twist the hands gently and return to a normal state from qigong state.

练功到此结束。

The end.

整体放松法
Whole Body Relaxation Method

整体放松法是将身体作为一个整体进行放松，要求目内视、意内想、耳内听、结合默念"松"字和存想放松部位感觉，从而达到放松的目的方法。习练时可以选取站、坐、卧、行中的任意一种，呼吸多采用自然呼吸或腹式呼吸。调心操作可以用心听自己念出的"松"字，也可以体会放松部位感觉。习练时操作3~5次，完整练习一遍的时间应该不少于10分钟。

This method relaxes the body as a whole. It requires inner visualization, inner meditation, inner listening and silent reading of the sound 'song' or experiencing the feeling of relaxation.

Posture: Standing, sitting, lying or walking.

Breathing: Natural or abdominal breathing.

Mental regulation can be performed by listening to the sound of 'Song' with heart or experiencing the feeling of relaxation of specific body parts. Repeat 3-5 times on each body part and it often takes at least 10 minutes to finish the whole set.

整体指的是外三合与内三合。外三合指的是形、气、神相合,内三合指的是肩髋相合、肘膝相合、手足相合。

The whole body includes three external unities and three internal unities. Three internal unities refer to body, qi and mind. Three external unties refer to shoulder-hip unity, elbow-knee unity and hand-foot unity.

整体放松时可以观想整个身体像一湖清水,丹田或命门就是湖的中央,细小的涟漪从丹田或命门轻轻荡起,一圈一圈地向外扩大,直至扩大到整个身体。随着涟漪扩大的过程,整个身体逐渐放松下来。就这样从内到外为一次,可以反复3~5次;也可以观想身体像一个空管,从上向下有水流通过,水流缓慢而均匀,随着水的不断流动,所过之处逐渐放松下来,从上到下为一次,可以反复3~5次;还可以观想身体像一个块海绵,干燥而且安静,有一股清泉从丹田或命门处开始向外流水,水被身体吸收,湿润的部分从内向外逐渐扩大,渐渐遍布全身,随着水分向外的扩散,身体逐渐放松下来。可以观想的场景还有很多,例如,可以观想身体是一块冰,从丹田或命门处开始融化,并逐渐向外扩散,直到整块冰都融化。

For whole body relaxation, you can visualize the body like a lake. Dantian or Mingmen is located at the center of the lake. Fine surface waves start to spread in circles from Dantian or Mingmen until they reach the entire body. Along with spreading of the surface wave, the whole body gradually relaxed from inward to outward. Repeat 3-5 times. Alternatively, you can visualize the body like a blank pipe to allow water to flow from top to bottom in slow even speed. Body parts along the pathway of water flow become relaxed, repeat 3-5 times. You can also visualize the body like a piece of dry sponge. Imagine a stream of spring water starts to flow out of Dantian or Mingmen. The body starts to absorb the water. The wet body parts are increased little by little. Gradually the entire body becomes wet. The body gradually relaxed along with the water flow. You can also visualize many other scenes, for example a piece of ice starting to melt from Dantian or Mingmen, gradually spreading until the ice completely melts.

整体放松法分为三步（或称三节），第一步整体放松，第二步意守丹田或命门，第三步玉液还丹。

There are three steps in this method: first, to relax by the sequence; second, focus mental consciousness on Dantian or Mingmen; and third, swallow saliva to Dantian.

整体放松法引导词一：

Guided words for whole body relaxation method (1):

现在开始练功了，停止工作，请安静下来，在正式练功前，先调整好姿势——调匀呼吸——保持平静的心态——

Before the practice of the whole body relaxation method, let's adjust our posture, breath naturally and keep a peaceful mind.

在放松的过程中，你要做的只是跟随口令，轻轻地体会放松的感觉。

What we need to do is to follow the word of command and

experience the feeling of relaxation.

现在开始练功：先把意识收回到体内，感觉身体像一湾湖水——湖水清澈见底——没有杂质——丹田就是湖的中心——我们从丹田开始放松——越来越松——越来越松——现在放松的感觉开始向周围扩散——像湖面的波纹一样——向外一圈一圈的扩散——随着波纹的扩散——身体的每一个部分都在放松——越来越松——越来越松——身体开始放松——身体越来越松——越来越松——身体完全放松——彻底放松——

Now let's start. Imagine our body as a lake — the lake water is so clear that you can see the bottom — there are no impurities — Dantian is located at the center of the lake — Dantian becomes relaxed — more relaxed — more and more relaxed — the relaxation starts to spread like the surface wave of the lake — spread outward in circles — each body part becomes relaxed along with spreading of the surface wave — more relaxed — more and more relaxed — our body starts to become relaxed — more relaxed — more and more relaxed — our body completely relaxed — thoroughly relaxed.

身体已经完全放松了，现在把意识轻轻地放到丹田——意守丹田——做3次深呼吸——

Now let's place our mental focus on Dantian, concentrate on Dantian and take 3 times of deep breathing.

现在把口中唾液分3次咽下，第一次——第二次——第三次——

Now let's swallow the saliva in three gulps, one — two —

three.

现在开始收功：轻轻地搓动两手——从练功状态慢慢地恢复到生活状态——

Now let's conclude: twist the hands gently and return to a normal state from qigong state.

练功到此结束。

The end.

整体放松法引导词二：

Guided words for whole body relaxation method (2):

现在开始练功了，停止工作，请安静下来，在正式练功前，先调整好姿势——调匀呼吸——保持平静的心态——

Before the practice of the whole body relaxation method, let's adjust our posture, breath naturally and keep a peaceful mind.

在放松的过程中，你要做的只是跟随口令，轻轻地体会放松的感觉。

What we need to do is to follow the word of command and experience the feeling of relaxation.

现在开始练功：先把意识收回到体内，感觉身体像一块冰——这块冰晶莹剔透——没有杂质——丹田就是这块冰的中心——从丹田开始变得温暖——越来越温暖——越来越温暖——这里的冰已经开始融化——逐渐融化——随着冰的融化丹田开始放松——越来越松——越来越松——现在这股暖流开始向周围扩散——温暖的范围开始扩大——融化的范围开始扩大——越来越大——越来越大——随着暖流的扩大身体越来越松——越来越松——越来越松——整块冰都融化了——变成一汪清水——身体完全放松了——彻底放松了——

Now let's start. Image our body as a piece of ice — crystal and clear — there are no impurities — Dantian is located at the center of this lake — the warm sensation starts from Dantian — warmer — warmer and warmer — now the ice starts to melt — melts little by little — the margins of the ice (our body) become relaxed — more relaxed — more and more relaxed — now the warm sensation spreads — warming area is increased little by little — bigger area — bigger and bigger area — our body becomes relaxed — more relaxed — more and more relaxed — the ice melted and turned into a stretch of clear water-- our body completely relaxed — thoroughly relaxed.

身体已经完全放松了, 现在把意识轻轻地放到丹田——意守丹田——做3次深呼吸——

Now let's place our mental focus on Dantian, concentrate on Dantian and take 3 times of deep breathing.

现在把口中唾液分3次咽下, 第一次——第二次——第三次——。

Now let's swallow the saliva in three gulps, one — two — three.

现在开始收功: 轻轻地搓动两手——从练功状态慢慢地恢

复到生活状态——

Now let's conclude: twist the hands gently and return to a normal state from qigong state.

练功到此结束。

The end.

倒行放松法
Reversed Relaxation Method

倒行放松法的操作与以上放松方法大致相同,只是各部位放松的顺序与以上方法相反。其规律一般为从脚到头,从外向内。但按顺序放松后,仍需把气引导丹田并将津液分3次咽下。

This method is almost same as the above-mentioned relaxation exercise, only in an opposite sequence. It's done from feet to the head and from exterior to interior. However, qi still needs to be guided to Dantian and saliva needs to be swallowed in three gulps after relaxation.

倒行松通法的操作顺序:

The sequence of reversed relaxing and unblocking method is as follows:

脚→踝关节→小腿→膝关节→大腿→髋关节→腰腹→胸背→手→腕关节→前臂→肘关节→上臂→肩→颈→头

Feet → ankle joints → lower legs → knee joints → thighs → hip joints→ waist and abdomen→ chest and back→

hands→ wrist joints→ forearms→ elbow joints→ upper arms→ shoulders → neck→ head.

倒行三线放松法的操作顺序：

The sequences of reversed three-line relaxation method are as follows:

第一条线：止息点是中冲穴→十个手指→两手→两腕→两前臂→两肘→两上臂→两肩→颈部两侧→头部两侧

Line # 1: Zhongchong (PC 9) → ten fingers → hands → wrists → forearms → elbows → upper arms → shoulders → both sides of the neck → both sides of the head.

第二条线：止息点是隐白穴→十个脚趾→两脚→两小腿→两膝→两大腿前→腹部→胸部→颈前→面部

Line # 2: Yinbai (SP 1) → ten toes → feet→ lower legs → knees → front of the thighs → abdomen → chest → front of the neck → face.

第三条线：止息点是涌泉穴 → 两脚底 → 两足跟 → 小腿后→两膝窝→大腿后→腰部→背部→后颈→后脑部

Line # 3: Yongquan (KI 1) → soles→ heels → back of the lower legs → popliteal fossae→ back of the thighs → waist→ back→ back of the neck → occiput.

分段放松法（倒行）的操作顺序：

The sequence of segmental relaxation method is as follows:

下肢→上肢→腹→胸→头

Lower limbs → upper limbs → abdomen → chest→ head.

倒行整体放松法则改为由外向内开始放松。

The whole body relaxation starts from outside to inside.

倒行松通法引导词：

Guided words for revised relaxing and unblocking method:

现在开始练功了，停止工作，请安静下来，在正式练功前，让我们先调整好姿势——调匀呼吸——保持平静的心态——

Before the practice of reversed relaxing and unblocking method, let's adjust our posture, breath naturally and keep a peaceful mind.

在放松的过程中，你要做的只是跟随口令，轻轻地体会放松的感觉。

What we need to do is to follow the word of command and experience the feeling of relaxation.

现在开始练功：先把意识集中到脚上，脚部放松——
松——松——→脚踝放松——松——松——→小腿放松——
松——松——→膝关节放松——松——松——→大腿放松——
松——松——→臀部放松——松——松——→腰腹放松——
松——松——→胸背放松——松——松——→手部放松——
松——松——→手腕部放松——松——松——→前臂放松——
松——松——→肘部放松——松——松——→上臂放松——

松——松———→肩部放松——松——松———→颈部放松——
松——松———→头部放松——松——松——

Now let's start. Relax the feet — Song — Song → relax the ankles — Song — Song → relax the lower legs — Song — Song → relax the knee joints — Song — Song →relax the thighs — Song — Song → relax the buttocks — Song — Song →relax the waist and abdomen — Song — Song → relax the chest and back — Song — Song → relax the hands — Song — Song → relax the wrist joints — Song — Song → relax the forearms — Song — Song → relax the elbows — Song — Song → relax the upper arms — Song — Song → relax the shoulders — Song — Song → relax the neck — Song — Song → relax the head — Song — Song.

身体已经完全放松了,现在把意识轻轻地放到丹田——意守丹田——做3次深呼吸——

Now let's place our mental focus on Dantian, concentrate on Dantian and take 3 times of deep breathing.

现在把口中唾液分3次咽下,第一次——第二次——第三次——

Now let's swallow the saliva in three gulps, one — two — three.

现在开始收功:轻轻地搓动两手——从练功状态慢慢地恢复到生活状态——

Now let's conclude: twist the hands gently and return to a normal state from qigong state.

练功到此结束。

The end.

倒行三线放松法引导词：

Guided words for revised three-line relaxation method:

现在开始练功了，停止工作，请安静下来，在正式练功前，先调整好姿势——调匀呼吸——保持平静的心态——

Before the practice of relaxing and unblocking method, let's adjust our posture, breath naturally and keep a peaceful mind.

在放松的过程中，你要做的只是跟随口令，轻轻地体会放松的感觉。

What we need to do is to follow the word of command and experience the feeling of relaxation.

现在开始练功：

Now let's start.

第一条线：身体两边放松——先把意识集中到脚上，→中冲穴放松——松——松——手指放松——松——松——→手部放松——松——松——→手腕放松——松——松——→前臂放松——松——松——→肘部放松——松——松——→上臂放松——松——松——→肩膀放松——松——松——→颈部两侧放松——松——松——→头部两侧放松——松——松——

Line # 1: Relax both sides of the body. Place the mental focus on the feet. Relax Zhongchong (PC 9) —

Song — Song → relax the fingers — Song — Song → relax the hands — Song — Song → relax the wrists — Song — Song → relax the forearms — Song — Song → relax the elbows — Song — Song → relax the upper arms — Song — Song → relax the shoulders — Song — Song → relax both sides of the neck — relax both sides of the head — Song — Song.

第二条线：身体前面放松——先把意识集中到脚上→隐白穴放松——松——松——脚趾放松——松——松——→两脚放松——松——松——→小腿放松——松——松——→膝关节放松——松——松——→两大腿前放松——松——松——→腹部放松——松——松——→胸部放松——松——松——→脖子前面放松——松——松——→面部放松——松——松——

Line # 2: Relax front of the body. Place the mental focus on the feet. Relax Yinbai (SP 1) — Song — Song → relax the toes — Song — Song → relax the feet — Song — Song → relax the lower legs — Song — Song →relax the knee joints — Song — Song → relax the front of the thighs — Song — Song → relax the abdomen — Song — Song → relax the chest — Song — Song → relax the front of the neck — Song — Song →relax the face — Song — Song.

第三条线：身体后面放松——先把意识集中到脚上→涌泉放松——松——松——→脚底放松——松——松——→脚跟放松——松——松——→小腿后面放松——松——松——→两个膝窝放松——松——松——→大腿后面放松——松——松——→腰部放松——松——松——→背部放松——松——松——→脖子后面放松——松——松——→头的后部放松——松——松——

Line # 3: Relax back of the body. Place the mental focus on the feet. Relax Yongquan (KI 1) — Song — Song → relax the soles — Song — Song → relax the heels — Song — Song → relax the back of the lower legs — Song — Song → relax the popliteal fossae — Song — Song → relax the back of the thighs — Song — Song →relax the waist — Song — Song → relax the back — Song — Song → relax the back of the neck — Song — Song → relax the occiput — Song — Song.

身体已经完全放松了，现在把意识轻轻地放到丹田——意守丹田——做3次深呼吸——

Now let's place our mental focus on Dantian, concentrate on Dantian and take 3 times of deep breathing.

现在把口中唾液分3次咽下，第一次——第二次——第三次——

Now let's swallow the saliva in three gulps, one — two — three.

现在开始收功：轻轻地搓动两手——从练功状态慢慢地恢复到生活状态——

Now let's conclude: twist the hands gently and return to a normal state from qigong state.

练功到此结束。
The end.

倒行分段放松法引导词：
Guided words for revised segmental relaxation method:

现在开始练功了,停止工作,请安静下来,在正式练功前,先调整好姿势——调匀呼吸——保持平静的心态——

Before the practice of revised segmental relaxation method, let's adjust our posture, breath naturally and keep a peaceful mind.

在放松的过程中,你要做的只是跟随口令,轻轻地体会放松的感觉。

What we need to do is to follow the word of command and experience the feeling of relaxation.

现在开始练功:先把意识集中到下肢,下肢放松 ——松——松———→上肢放松——松——松———→腰腹部放松——松——松———→胸背部放松——松——松———→头部放松——松——松——

Now let's start. Relax the lower limbs — Song — Song → relax the upper limbs — Song — Song → relax the waist and abdomen — Song — Song → relax the chest and back —Song — Song → relax the head — Song — Song.

身体已经完全放松了,现在把意识轻轻地放到丹田——意守丹田——做3次深呼吸——

Now let's place our mental focus on Dantian, concentrate on Dantian and take 3 times of deep breathing.

现在把口中唾液分3次咽下,第一次——第二次——第三次——

Now let's swallow the saliva in three gulps, one — two — three.

现在开始收功：轻轻地搓动两手——从练功状态慢慢地恢复到生活状态——

Now let's conclude: twist the hands gently and return to a normal state from qigong state.

练功到此结束。

The end.

倒行整体放松法引导词一：

Guided words for revised whole body relaxation method (1):

现在开始练功了，停止工作，请安静下来，在正式练功前，先调整好姿势——调匀呼吸——保持平静的心态——

Before the practice of revised whole body relaxation method, let's adjust our posture, breath naturally and keep a peaceful mind.

在放松的过程中，你要做的只是跟随口令，轻轻地体会放松的感觉。

What we need to do is to follow the word of command and experience the feeling of relaxation.

现在开始练功：先把意识收回到体内，身体像一湾湖水——湖水清澈见底——没有杂质——身体边缘开始放松——越来越松——越来越松——现在放松的感觉开始向湖心扩散——像湖面的波纹一样———圈一圈的向丹田扩散——逐渐扩散——所有放松的感觉都扩散到丹田——身体越来越松——

越来越松——身体的每一个部分都在放松——越来越松——越来越松——身体完全放松——彻底放松了——

Now let's start. Imagine our body as a lake — the lake water is so clear that you can see the bottom — there are no impurities — the margins of the lake (our body) start to relax — more relaxed — more and more relaxed — now the feeling of relaxation spread to the middle of the lake — just like the surface wave of the lake — spread to Dantian in circles — spread little by little — all feelings of relaxation spread to Dantian — our body becomes more relaxed — more and more relaxed — each body part becomes relaxed — more relaxed — more and more relaxed — our body completely relaxed — thoroughly relaxed.

身体已经完全放松了，现在把意识轻轻地放到丹田——意守丹田——做3次深呼吸——

Now let's place our mental focus on Dantian, concentrate on Dantian and take 3 times of deep breathing.

现在把口中唾液分3次咽下，第一次——第二次——第三次——

Now let's swallow the saliva in three gulps, one — two — three.

现在开始收功：轻轻地搓动两手——从练功状态慢慢地恢复到生活状态——

Now let's conclude: twist the hands gently and return to a normal state from qigong state.

练功到此结束。

The end.

整体放松法引导词二：

现在开始练功了，停止工作，请安静下来，在正式练功前，先调整好姿势——调匀呼吸——保持平静的心态——

Before the practice of revised whole body relaxation method, let's adjust our posture, breath naturally and keep a peaceful mind.

在放松的过程中，你要做的只是跟随口令，轻轻地体会放松的感觉。

What we need to do is to follow the word of command and experience the feeling of relaxation.

现在开始练功：先把意识收回到体内，感觉身体像一块冰——这块冰晶莹剔透——没有杂质——从身体的边缘开始变得温暖——越来越温暖——越来越温暖——这里的冰已经开始融化——逐渐融化——随着冰的融化身体的边缘开始放松——越来越松——越来越松——现在这股暖流开始向体内扩散——温暖的范围逐渐扩大——越来越大——越来越大——身体开始放松——越来越松——越来越松——一直放松到丹田——整个身体都融化了——变成一汪清水——身体完全放松了——彻底放松了——

Now let's start. Image our body as a piece of ice — crystal and clear — there are no impurities — the margins of the ice (our body) start to become warm — warmer — warmer and warmer — now the ice starts to melt — melts little by little — the margins of the ice (our body) become relaxed — more relaxed — more and more relaxed — now the warm sensation spread inside the body — the warm amplitude is increased little by little — bigger amplitude — bigger and bigger amplitude — our body becomes relaxed — more relaxed — more and more relaxed — the Dantian relaxed — the whole body melted — and turned into a stretch of clear water — our body completely relaxed — thoroughly relaxed.

身体已经完全放松了，现在把意识轻轻地放到丹田——意守丹田——做3次深呼吸——

Now let's place our mental focus on Dantian, concentrate on Dantian and take 3 times of deep breathing.

现在把口中唾液分3次咽下，第一次——第二次——第三次——

Now let's swallow the saliva in three gulps, one — two — three.

现在开始收功：轻轻地搓动两手——从练功状态慢慢地恢复到生活状态——

Now let's conclude: twist the hands gently and return to a normal state from qigong state.

练功到此结束。

The end.

振颤放松法
Shaking/trembling Relaxation Method

振颤放松法是通过振颤、抖动使全身放松的一种方法。振颤放松法习练时站、坐、行均可。全身振颤时以站式较容易操作,局部振颤时,站、坐两种姿势较为容易操作。振颤的幅度较小,频率相对较快,可以全身振颤,也可以局部振颤。抖动的幅度相对较大,频率相对较慢,可以全身抖动,也可以局部抖动。

This method relaxes the body by trembling and shaking. It can be done in standing, sitting or walking. It's easy to perform the whole body trembling in standing. As for local trembling, it's easy to perform in a standing or sitting position. The trembling is small in amplitude and high in frequency. Trembling can involve the whole body or localized body parts. Shaking is bigger in amplitude but lower in frequency. Likewise, shaking can involve the whole body or specific body parts.

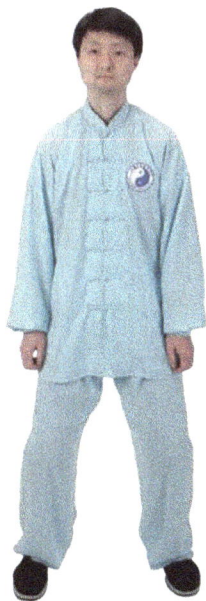

抖动放松图　Shaking relaxation method

振颤、抖动时身体要放松，各关节似有弹性，有节奏，不要僵硬。全身抖动时，可以把踝关节作为起点和发力点。逐渐向上扩散，最后带动全身抖动。也可以把丹田或命门作为起点，和发力点（抖动放松图）。逐渐向全身扩散，最后带动全身抖动。在抖动过程中要保持身体的中正，不要歪斜。抖动要自然发生，抖动的幅度与频率都要顺其自然，不要刻意去抖。向全身扩散的过程也要顺其自然，遇到身体某处较为紧张，难以放松，一时抖不起来，不要着急，可以先做其他部位的抖动，耐心等待一会就好了。

The body needs to be relaxed during trembling or shaking. Make sure the shaking or trembling of joints to be elastic or rhythmic. The whole body shaking can start or exert force from the ankle joints and gradually spread upward. Alternatively, it can start or exert force from Dantian or Mingmen. It's essential to keep the body upright during shaking. In addition, it's important not to force yourself to shake or tremble but follow the natural amplitude and frequency. In case it's hard to relax some body parts, just be patient and shake or tremble other body parts first.See the Fig of shaking relaxation method.

振颤、抖动放松法一般采用自然呼吸。
This method uses natural breathing.

心理操作较为简单，可以体会身体在颤动、抖动过程中逐渐放松的感觉。也可以意想全身如网状通透，将体内病气、浊气随着抖动向下排出。全身振颤、抖动后，静立3~6分钟。

As for mental regulation, just experience the feeling of relaxation during shaking or trembling. You can also imagine the whole body like a transparent net and you are shaking to discharging pathogens or turbid qi out of the body. After shaking or trembling, stand still for 3-6 minutes.

全身抖动法引导词：

Guided words for whole body shaking method:

现在开始练功了，停止工作，请安静下来，在正式练功前，先调整好姿势——调匀呼吸——保持平静的心态——

Before the practice of the whole body shaking method, let's adjust our posture, breath naturally and keep a peaceful mind.

在放松的过程中，你要做的只是跟随口令，轻轻地体会抖动的感觉。

What we need to do is to follow the word of command and experience the feeling of shaking.

现在开始练功：先把意识收回到体内，身体开始放松——逐渐放松——越来越松——内心越来越平静——越来越平静——脚踝那里开始抖动——幅度逐渐增大——越来越大——越来越大——腿部也开始抖动了——幅度逐渐增大——越来越大——全身都在抖动——幅度逐渐增大——越来越大——就这样不停地抖———一直在抖———一直在抖——现在抖动的幅度开始减小了——逐渐减小——越来越小——越来越小——现在身体不抖了——身体恢复了原来的姿势——

Now let's start. Our body starts to relax — relax little by little — more and more relaxed — our mind becomes serene — more and more serene — the ankles start to shake — the shaking amplitude is increased little by little — bigger amplitude — bigger and bigger amplitude — the legs start to shake — the shaking amplitude is increased little by little — bigger amplitude — bigger and bigger amplitude — the whole body starts to shake — the shaking amplitude is increased little by little — bigger amplitude — constant shaking — keep shaking — still keep shaking — now the shaking amplitude is decreased little by little — smaller amplitude — smaller and smaller amplitude — now the body stops shaking — the body returns to normal position.

身体已经完全放松了，现在把意识轻轻地放到丹田——意守丹田——做3次深呼吸——

Now let's place our mental focus on Dantian, concentrate on Dantian and take 3 times of deep breathing.

现在把口中唾液分3次咽下，第一次——第二次——第三次——

Now let's swallow the saliva in three gulps, one — two — three.

现在开始收功：轻轻地搓动两手——从练功状态慢慢地恢复到生活状态——

Now let's conclude: twist the hands gently and return to a normal state from qigong state.

练功到此结束。

The end.

全身振颤法引导词：

Guided words for whole body trembling method:

现在开始练功了，停止工作，请安静下来，在正式练功前，先调整好姿势——调匀呼吸——保持平静的心态——

Before the practice of the whole body trembling method, let's adjust our posture, breath naturally and keep a peaceful mind.

在放松的过程中，你要做的只是跟随口令，轻轻地体会振颤的感觉。

What we need to do is to follow the word of command and experience the feeling of trembling.

现在开始练功：先把意识收回到体内，身体开始放松——逐渐放松——越来越松——内心越来越平静——越来越平静——左手开始颤动——很细微的颤动——颤动越来越明显——越来越明显——幅度逐渐增大——越来越大——越来越大——整个手臂也开始颤动了——幅度逐渐增大——越来越大——全身都在颤动——幅度逐渐增大——越来越大——就这样不停地颤——一直在颤——一直在颤——现在颤动的幅度开始减小了——逐渐减小——越来越小——越来越小——现在身体不颤了——身体恢复了原来的姿势——

Now let's start. Our body starts to relax---relax little by little — more and more relaxed — our mind becomes serene — more and more serene — the left hand starts to tremble — very subtle trembling — more and more obvious trembling — more and more trembling — the trembling amplitude is increased little by little — bigger amplitude — bigger and bigger amplitude — the whole arm starts to tremble — the trembling amplitude is increased little by little — bigger amplitude — bigger and bigger amplitude — constant trembling — keep trembling — still keep trembling — the trembling amplitude is decreased little by little — smaller amplitude — smaller and smaller amplitude — now the body stops trembling — the body returns to normal position.

身体已经完全放松了，现在把意识轻轻地放到丹田——意守丹田——做3次深呼吸——

Now let's place our mental focus on Dantian, concentrate on Dantian and take 3 times of deep breathing.

现在把口中唾液分3次咽下，第一次——第二次——第三次——

Now let's swallow the saliva in three gulps, one — two — three.

现在开始收功：轻轻地搓动两手——从练功状态慢慢地恢复到生活状态——

Now let's conclude: twist the hands gently and return to a normal state from qigong state.

练功到此结束。
The end.

拍打放松法
Tapping Relaxation Method

拍打放松法是采用拍打的方式，由外而内放松的一种方法。拍打的部位常常是经络循行的部位。拍打时五指自然弯曲，形成空心拳，叩击时轻柔而有弹性，切忌用力。叩击时手腕放松，随呼气叩击。

This method is to relax the body from outside to inside by tapping the meridians. Relax the wrist, breathe out and use naturally curled fingers (an empty fist) to tap gently (do not use too much force).

拍打法一　经络拍打线路

Method # 1 Tap along the meridians

叩击穴位依次为：百会→耳门→天牖→天髎→肩髎→消泺→天井→外关→阳池→中渚→外关→中冲→劳宫→大陵→内关→曲泽→天泉

Tap along the sequence of the following points: Baihui (DU 20) → Ermen (SJ 21) → Tianyou (SJ 16) → Tiaoliao (SJ 15) → Jianliao (SJ 14) → Xiaopo (SJ 12) → Tianjing (SJ 10) → Waiguan (SJ 5) → Yangchi (SJ 4) →Zhongzhu (SJ 3) → Waiguan (SJ 5) → Zhongchong (PC 9) → Laogong (PC 8) → Daling (PC 7) → Neiguan (PC 6) → Quze (PC 3) → Tianquan (PC 2)

百会→阳白→四白→地仓→缺盆→乳根→天枢→髀关→伏兔→足三里→丰隆→解溪→内庭→历兑

Baihui (DU 20) → Yangbai (GB 14) → Sibai (ST 2) → Quepen (ST 12) → Rugen (ST 18) → Tianshu (ST 25) → Biguan (ST 31) → Futu (ST 32) → Zusanli (ST 36) → Fenglong (ST 40) → Jiexi (ST 41) → Neiting (ST 44) → Lidui (ST 45)

百会→天柱→肾俞→胞肓→承扶→殷门→委中→承山→昆

仑→束骨→至阴

Baihui (DU 20) → Tianzhu (BL 10) → Shenshu (BL 23) → Baohuang (BL 53) → Chengfu (BL 36) → Yinmen (BL 37) → Weizhong (BL 40) → Chengshan (BL 57) → Kunlun (BL 60) → Shugu (BL 65) → Zhiyin (BL 67)

拍打法二　简易拍打

Movement # 2 Simple tapping

采用站式或坐式，从上到下依次分段进行有步律的拍打放松。拍打路线：

Simple tapping from the head to foot can be done in a standing or sitting position. Be sure to tap with a rhythm.

左肩外侧→左上臂外侧→左肘关节外侧→左小臂外侧→左手腕外侧→左手背 (拍打放松图 1~6)。

Tapping route: Lateral left shoulder→lateral left upper arm → lateral left elbow → lateral left forearm → lateral left wrist → dorsum of the left hand. (simple tapping 1–6)

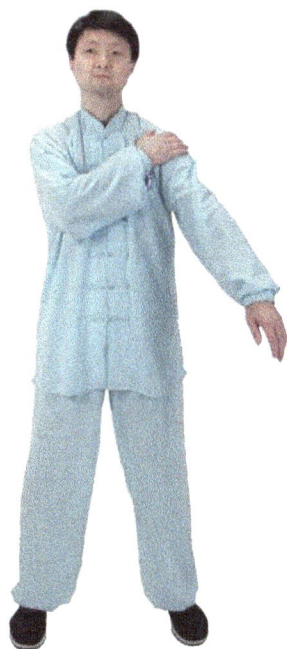

拍打放松图 1　Simple tapping 1

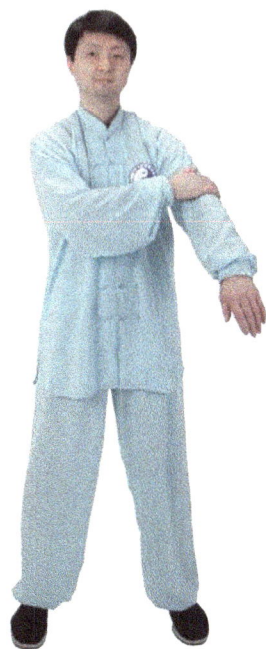

拍打放松图 2　Simple tapping 2

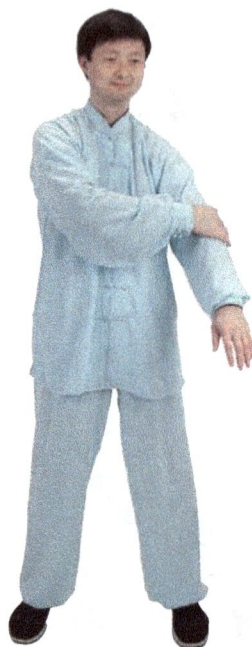

拍打放松图 3　　Simple tapping 3

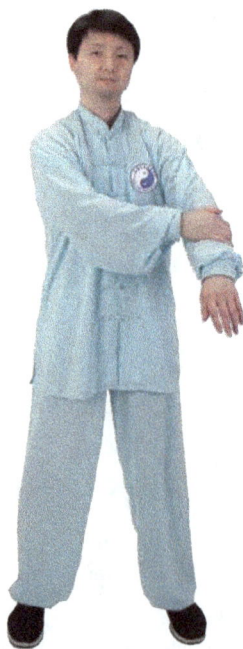

拍打放松图 4　　Simple tapping 4

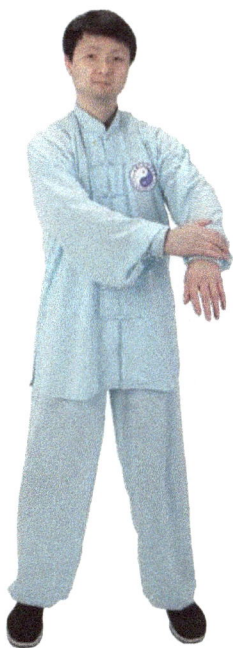

拍打放松图5　Simple tapping 5

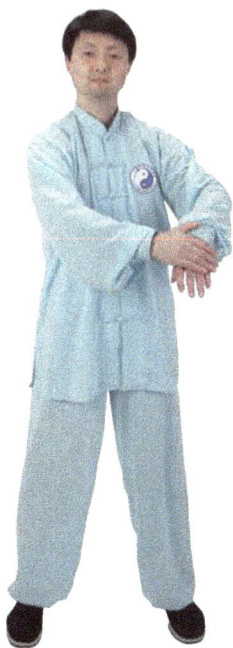

拍打放松图6　Simple tapping 6

左肩内侧→左上臂内侧→左肘关节内侧→左小臂内侧→左

手腕内侧→左手掌(拍打放松图7~12)。

Medial left shoulder → medial left upper arm → medial left elbow → medial left forearm → medial left wrist → left palm. (simple tapping 7–12)

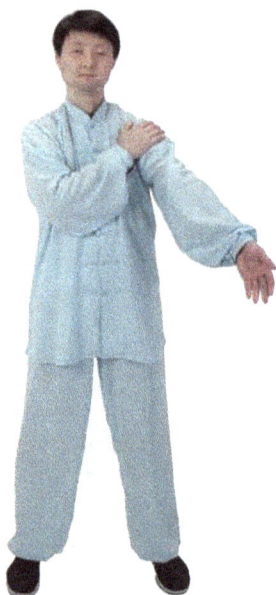

拍打放松图7　Simple tapping 7

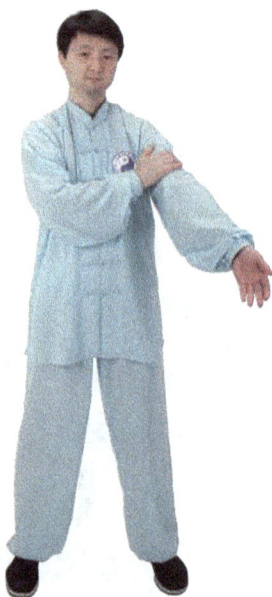

拍打放松图8　Simple tapping 8

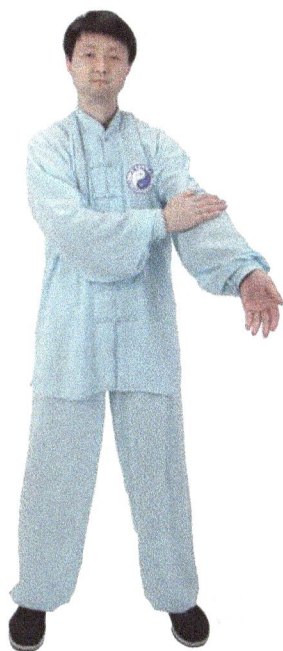

拍打放松图 9　Simple tapping 9

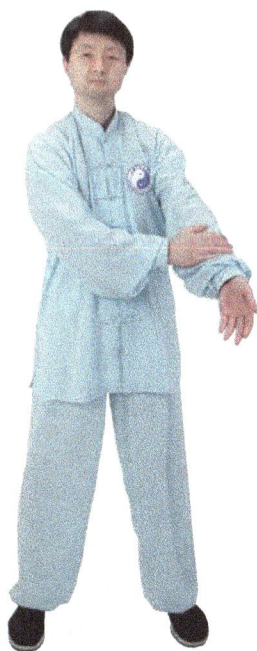

拍打放松图 10　Simple tapping 10

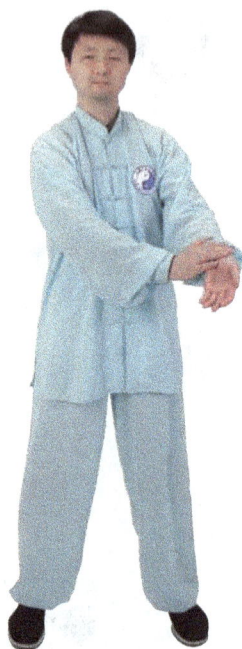

拍打放松图11　Simple tapping 11

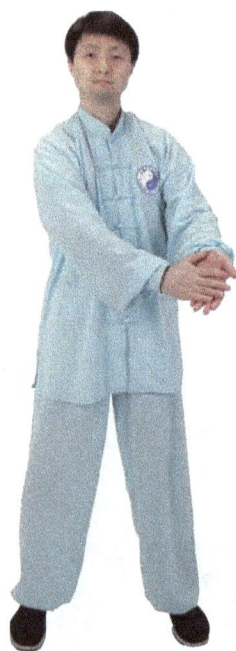

拍打放松图12　Simple tapping 12

右肩外侧→右上臂外侧→右肘关节外侧→右小臂外侧→右

手腕外侧→右手背(拍打放松图13~18)。

Lateral right shoulder → lateral right upper arm → lateral right elbow → lateral right arm → lateral right wrist → dorsum of the right hand.(simple tapping 13–18)

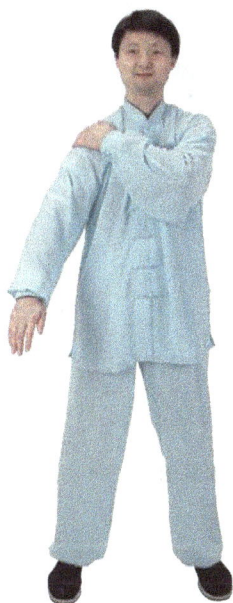

拍打放松图 13　Simple tapping 13

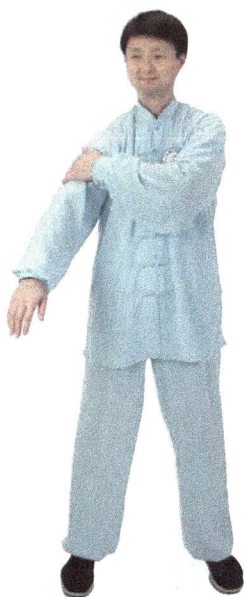

拍打放松图 14　Simple tapping 14

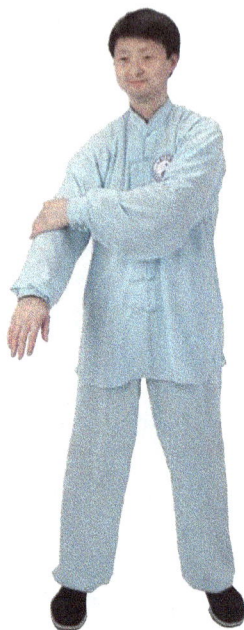

拍打放松图 15　Simple tapping 15

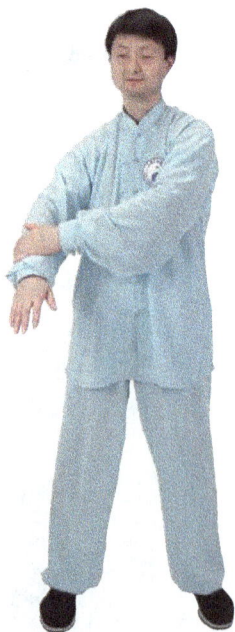

拍打放松图 16　Simple tapping 16

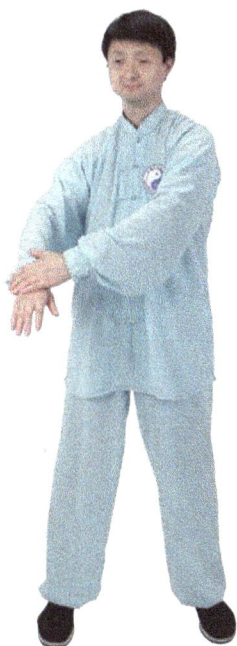

拍打放松图 17　Simple tapping 17

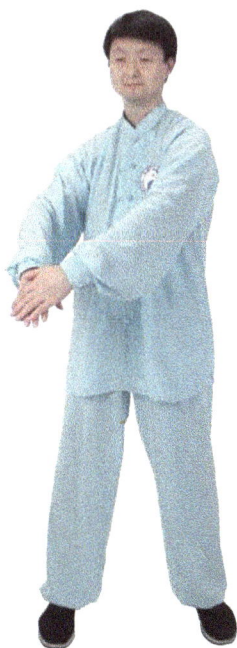

拍打放松图 18　Simple tapping 18

右肩内侧→右上臂内侧→右肘关节内侧→右小臂内侧→右

手腕内侧→右手掌(拍打放松图19~24)。

　　Medial right shoulder → medial right upper arm → medial right elbow → medial right forearm → medial right wrist → right palm.(simple tapping 19–24)

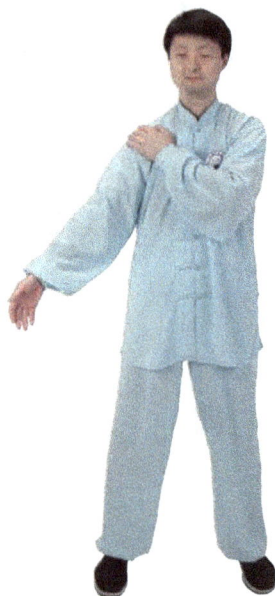

拍打放松图19　Simple tapping 19

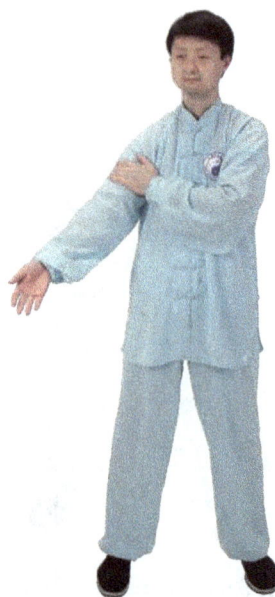

拍打放松图20　Simple tapping 20

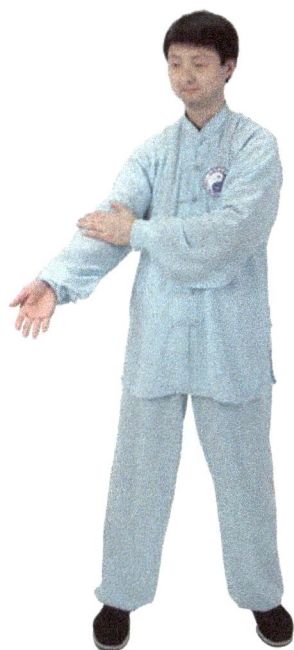

拍打放松图 21   Simple tapping 21

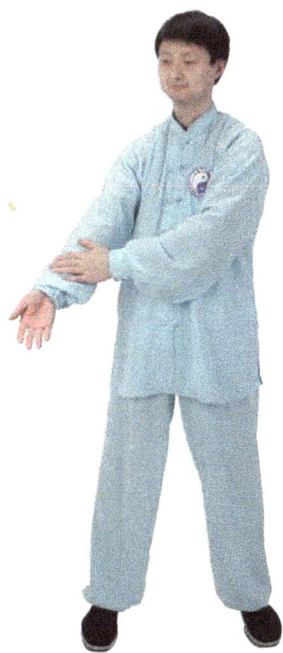

拍打放松图 22   Simple tapping 22

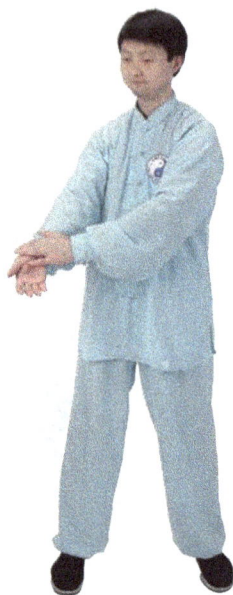

拍打放松图23　Simple tapping 23

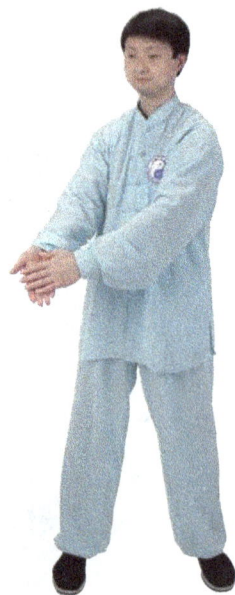

拍打放松图24　Simple tapping 24

　　两肋→两胯→两大腿外侧→两膝外侧→两小腿外侧→两踝外侧→两脚外侧 (拍打放松图25~31)。

Two ribs → two hip joints → bilateral sides of the thighs → bilateral sides of the knees → bilateral sides of the lower legs → bilateral sides of the malleolus → bilateral sides of the foots.(simple tapping 25–31)

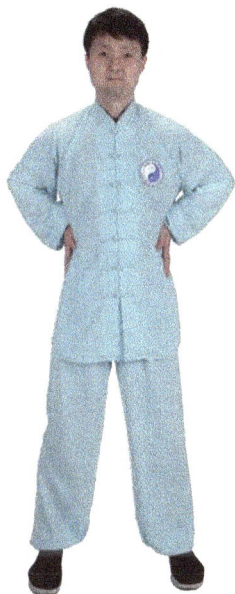

拍打放松图25　Simple tapping 25

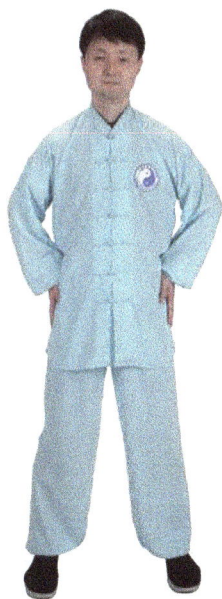

拍打放松图26　Simple tapping 26

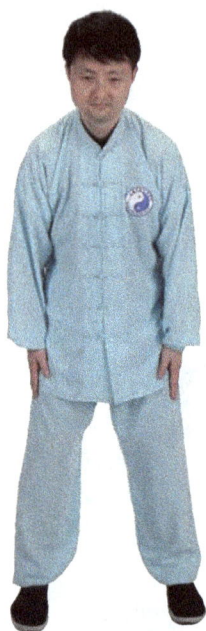

拍打放松图27　Simple tapping 27

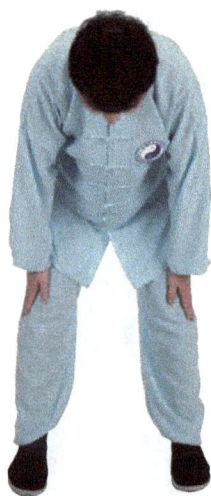

拍打放松图28　Simple tapping 28

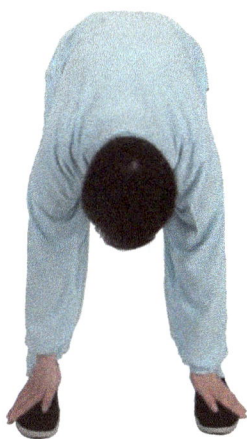

拍打放松图29　Simple tapping 29　　　拍打放松图30　Simple tapping 30

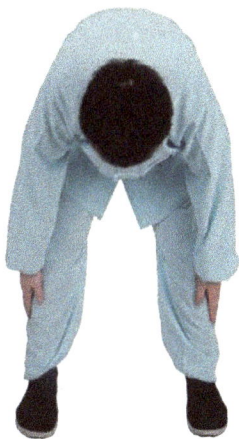

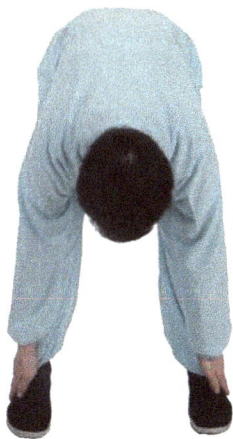

拍打放松图31　Simple tapping 31

　　胸→上腹→小腹→大腿前面→膝关节前面→小腿前面→踝关节前面→脚背(拍打放松图32~39)。

　　Chest → upper abdomen → lower abdomen → front of the thighs → front of the knee joints → front of the lower legs → front of the ankle joint → dorsum of the feet.(simple tapping 32–39)

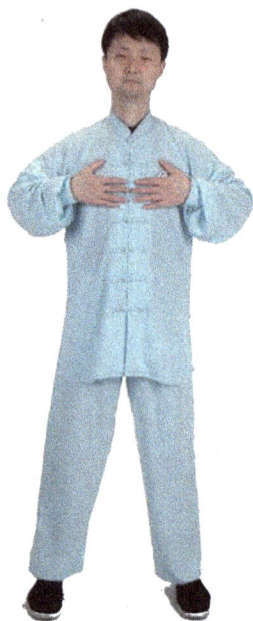

拍打放松图 32　Simple tapping 32

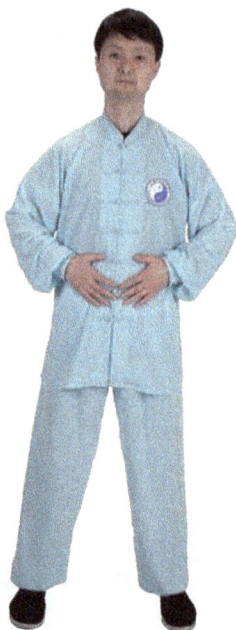

拍打放松图 33　Simple tapping 33

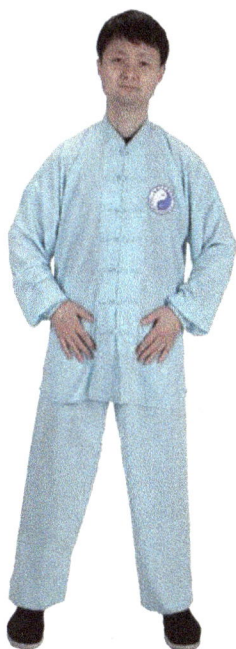

拍打放松图 34　Simple tapping 34

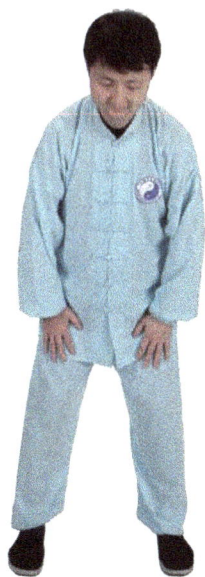

拍打放松图 35　Simple tapping 35

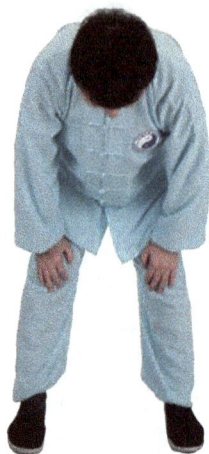

拍打放松图 36　　Simple tapping 36

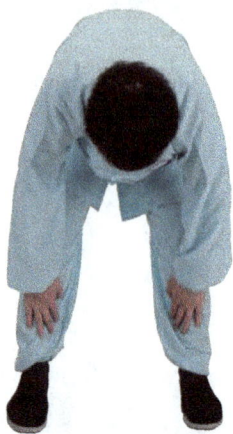

拍打放松图 37　　Simple tapping 37

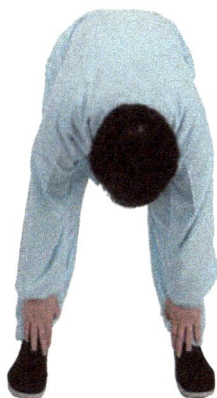

拍打放松图 38　Simple tapping 38

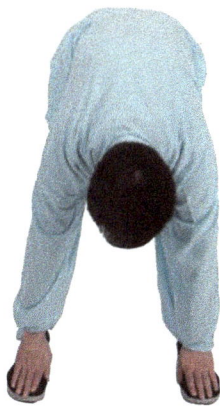

拍打放松图 39　Simple tapping 39

腰→臀→大腿后面→膝关节后面→小腿后面→足跟(拍打放松图40~45)。

Waist → buttocks → back of the thighs→ back of the knee joints → back of the lower legs → heels.(simple tapping 40–45)

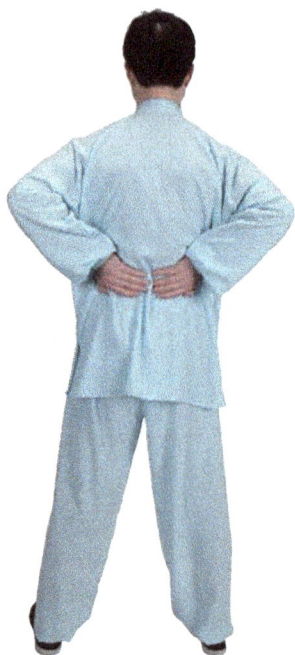

拍打放松图 40　Simple tapping 40

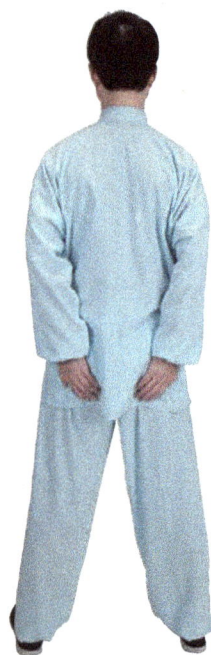

拍打放松图 41　Simple tapping 41

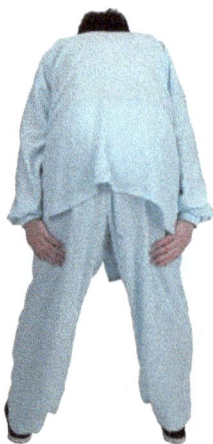

拍打放松图 42　Simple tapping 42

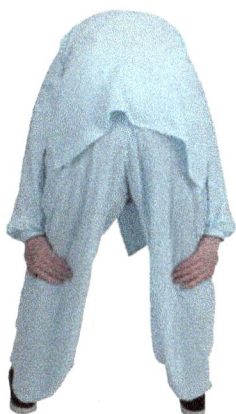

拍打放松图43　Simple tapping 43

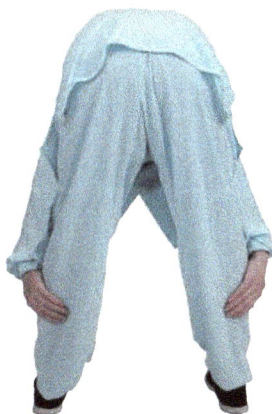

拍打放松图44　Simple tapping 44

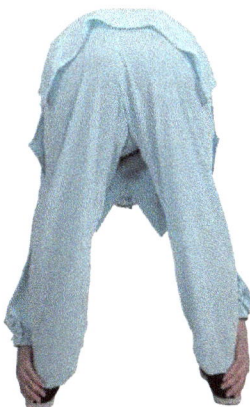

拍打放松图45　Simple tapping 45

坐式与站式原理相同。

Sit and stand for the same principle.

现在开始练功了，停止工作，请安静下来，在正式练功前，先调整好姿势——调匀呼吸——保持平静的心态——

Before practice, let's adjust our posture, breath naturally and keep a peaceful mind.

在放松的过程中，你要做的只是跟随口令，轻轻地体会放松的感觉。

During the relaxing process, you only need to follow the word of command and experience the relaxation.

现在开始轻轻地拍打——

Now let's start.

自然呼吸，体会被拍打部位的逐渐放松，意想体内的病气、浊气在拍打过程中向下移动到肢体末端，进而排出体外。

Breathe naturally. Experience the relaxing sensation in the tapping area. During tapping, use you mind to move the pathogenic and turbid qi down to four extremities and remove out of the body.

身体已经完全放松了，现在把意识轻轻地放到丹田——意守丹田——做3次深呼吸——

Now let's place our mental focus on Dantian, concentrate on Dantian and take 3 times of deep breathing.

现在把口中唾液分3次咽下，第一次——第二次——第三次——

Now let's swallow the saliva in three gulps, one — two — three.

现在开始收功：轻轻地搓动两手——从练功状态慢慢地恢复到生活状态——

Now let's conclude: twist the hands gently and return to a normal state from qigong state.

练功到此结束。

The end.

功后动作
Movements after conclusion

1. 浴面
1. Wash the face

搓热两手，以中指沿鼻两侧，自下而上，带动其他手指，搓到额部向两侧分开，经两颊而下，计6次。可使面部气血流畅，预防感冒（功后动作图1~3）。

Twist the hands until they become warm. Use the middle finger to guide other fingers to rub from bottom to top along bilateral sides of the nose. Separate the hands at the forehead and then rub down along the cheeks. Repeat 9 times. This movement can circulate qi and blood in the face and prevent common colds. (movements after

conclusion 1–3)

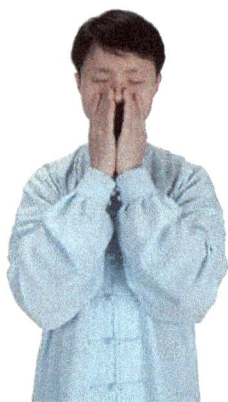

功后动作图1　movements after conclusion 1

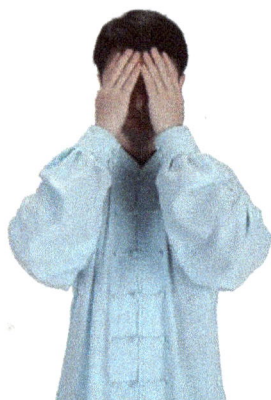

功后动作图2　movements after conclusion 2

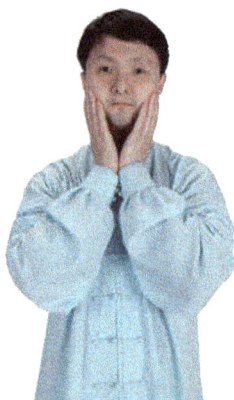

功后动作图3　movements after conclusion 3

2. 鸣鼓

2. Make the drum sound

　　两手掩耳，然后以示指压在中指之上，滑下来轻弹后脑部，计6次。经常做可以预防头昏耳鸣等（功后动作图4~5）。

Cover the ears: Cover the ear with the palms of both hands and count 9 times of breathing through the nose. Then place the index fingers on top of the middle fingers and firmly snap the index finger off the middle finger and onto the back of the head making a drumming sound. The tapping should be repeated for a total of 24 times. This movement can prevent and treat dizziness and tinnitus. (movements after conclusion 4–5)

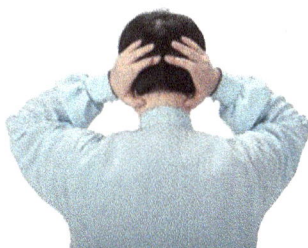

功后动作图4　movements after conclusion 4

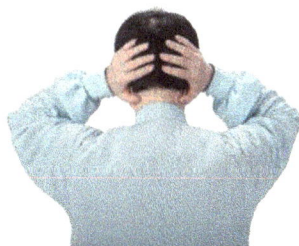

功后动作图5　movements after conclusion 5

3. 左顾右盼
Look right and left

两眼先向前平视，随着头颈转向左，两目斜视左肩，然后头颈转向右，两目斜视右肩，左右各6次。能舒松颈背，操作时须缓缓而行（功后动作图6~7）。

Look straight ahead first, then turn the head and neck to left, focus the eyes on the left shoulder. After this, turn the head and neck to right and focus the eyes on the right shoulder. Repeat 6 times on each side. This can relax the neck and back. (Caution) This movement should be done slowly. (movements after conclusion 6–7)

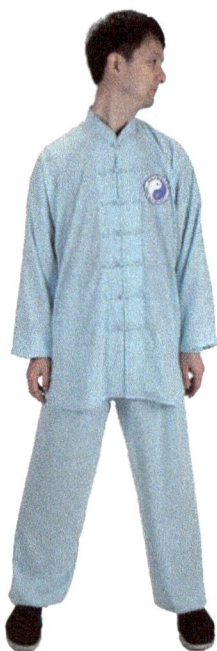

功后动作图6
movements after conclusion 6

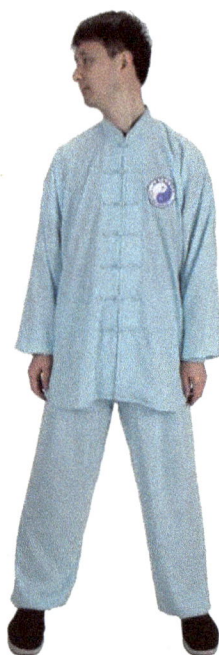

功后动作图7
movements after conclusion 7

4. 擦腰
Rub the lower back

搓热两手，擦背下腰软处，左右手上下交替6次。可防治腰背酸痛（功后动作图8~9）。

Twist the hands until they become warm. Then rub the lower back with both hands (up and down alternately) for a total of 24 times. This movement can prevent and treat lower back pain. (movements after conclusion 8–9)

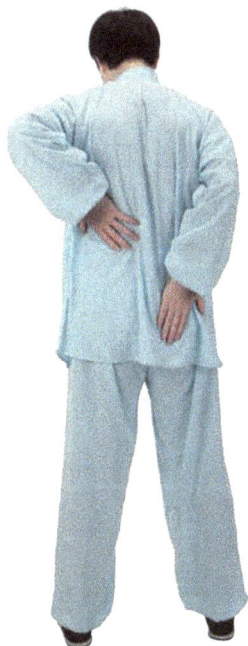

功后动作图 8
movements after conclusion 8

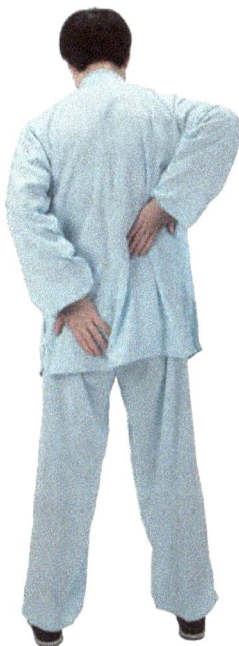

功后动作图 9
movements after conclusion 9

5. 双手齐伸开
Extend the hands

双手握固（握拳，大拇指握在四指之内，见功后动作图 10）

Place the thumbs of both hands under the other four fingers. (movements after conclusion 10)

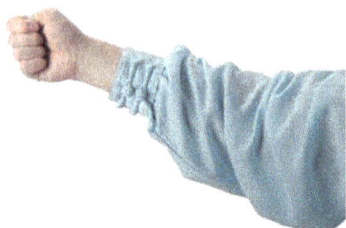

功后动作图 10
movements after conclusion 10

　　拳眼向上，放近胸前，再向左右两侧徐徐拉开，计6次。可增强肺气，减轻胸闷（功后动作图11~12）。

make the holes of the fists (space between the thumb and index finger) upward and place the fists close to the chest. Then slowly open up the hands to both sides for a total of 24 times. This movement can enhance lung qi and relieve chest tightness. (movements after conclusion 11–12)

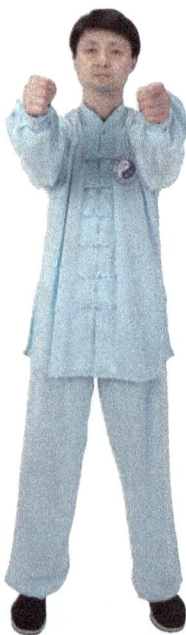

功后动作图 11
movements after conclusion 11

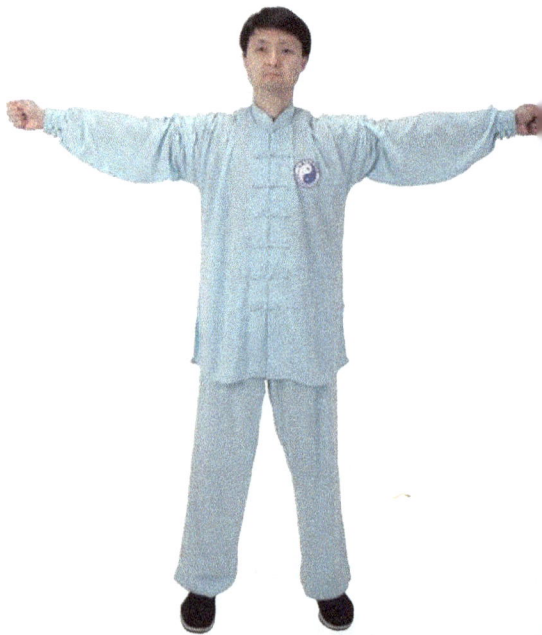

功后动作图 12
movements after conclusion 12

6. 双转辘轳

Rotate the winch

双手握固, 平伸, 拳心向下, 向上前方伸展, 如摇转辘轳一样, 计6次。可舒展上肢关节 (功后动作图13~16)。

Place the thumbs of both hands under the other four fingers and make the palmar side of the fists downward. Then extend the fists upward and forward like rotating a winch for a total of 12 times. This movement can stretch the upper limb joints. (movements after conclusion 13–16)

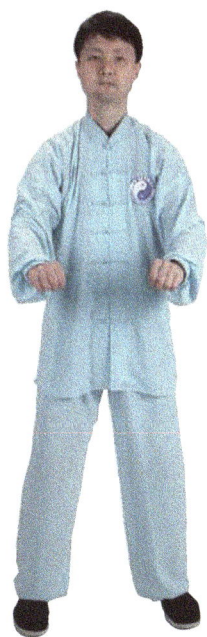

功后动作图13
movements after conclusion 13

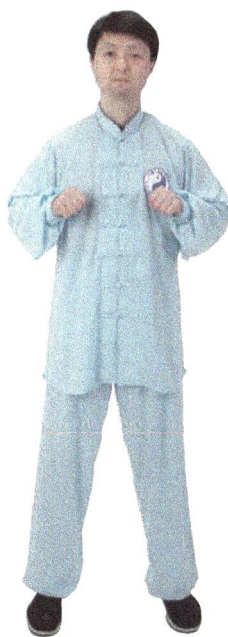

功后动作图14
movements after conclusion 14

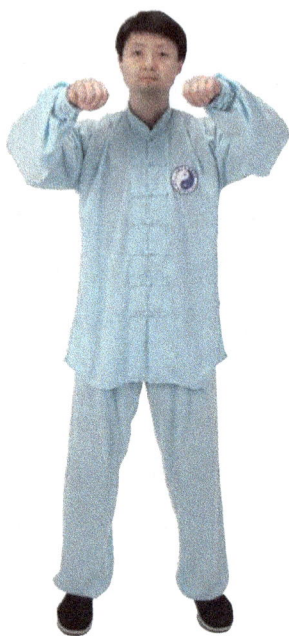

功后动作图 15   movements after conclusion 15

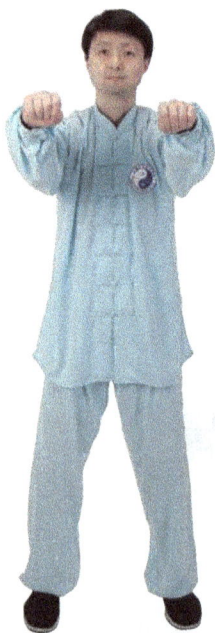

功后动作图 16   movements after conclusion 16

7. 左右托天
Lift the sky with both hands

以一手叉腰，一手轻慢提起，过双眉时翻手，掌心向上，托过头顶，伸直手臂；同时两目注视手背，两手交替进行各5次。能调理脾胃，增强消化，舒展上肢关节（功后动作图17~23）。

Place one hand on the side of the waist, slowly lift the other hand and turn over the hand (palms upward) at the level of the eyebrows. Lift the hand up above the top of the head and extend the arm. Focus the eyes on the dorsum of the hand. Repeat 5 times on each hand. This movement can regulate the spleen and stomach, increase digestion and stretch upper limb joints. (movements after conclusion 17–23)

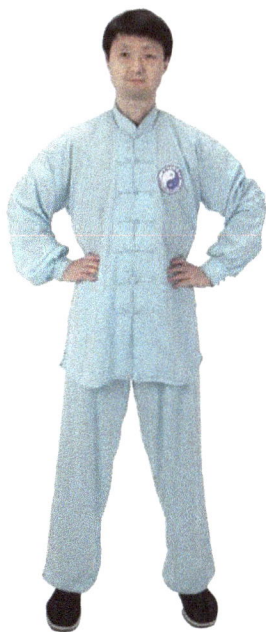

功后动作图17
movements after conclusion 17

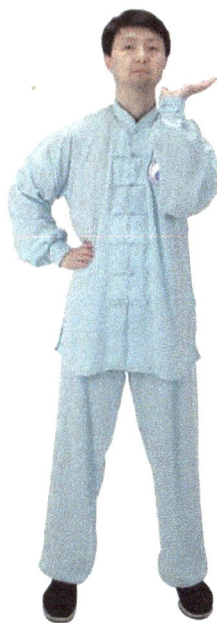

功后动作图18
movements after conclusion 18

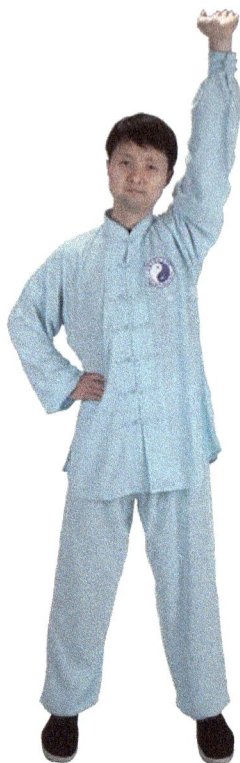

功后动作图 19　movements after conclusion 19

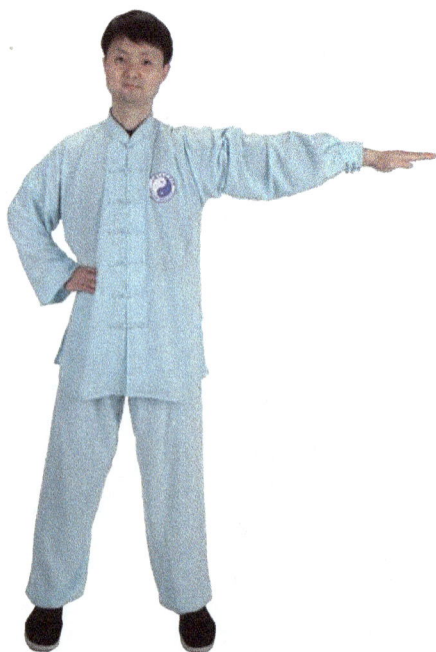

功后动作图 20　movements after conclusion 20

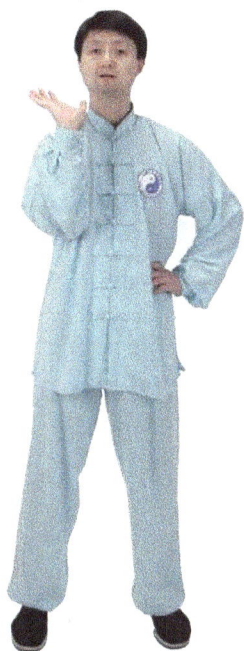

功后动作图21
movements after conclusion 21

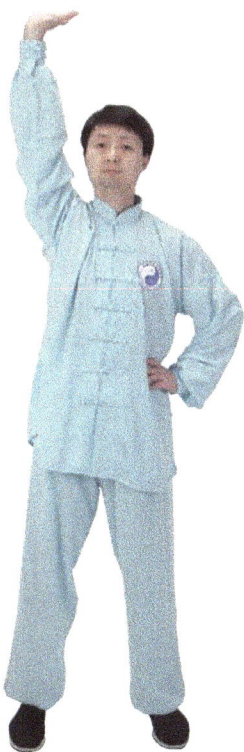

功后动作图22
movements after conclusion 22

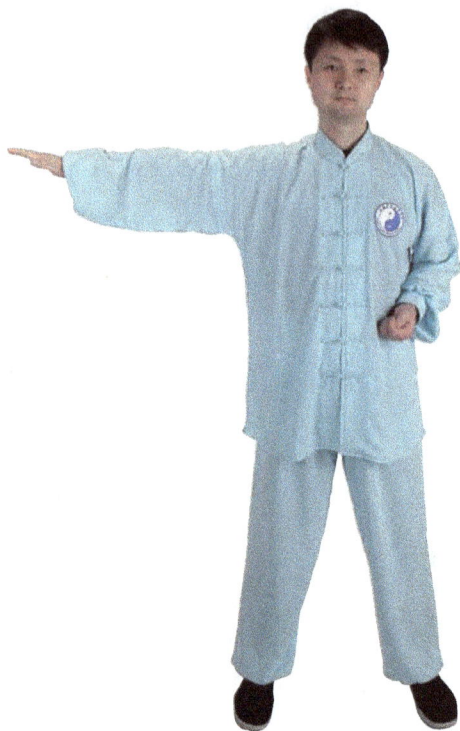

功后动作图23　movements after conclusion 23

8. 双手攀足
Grasping the feet with hands

伸直两腿，搁在前面，上身向前俯，双手去攀足，以逐渐能攀到前脚心为度：每攀一次，轻拍大腿二三下，做7次。可舒松筋骨，增强腹肌，固肾强腰（功后动作图24~26）。

Extend the legs, bend the upper body forward, use both hands to grasp the feet (gradually touch the soles) and then tap the thigh 2-3 times. Repeat the procedure 7 times. This movement can relax the tendons and bones, strengthen abdominal muscles, benefit the kidney and consolidate the waist. (movements after conclusion 24–26)

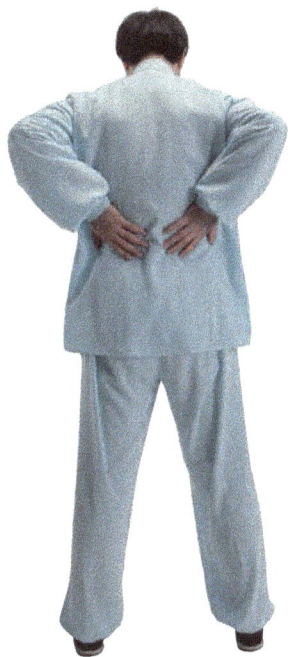

功后动作图24
movements after conclusion 24

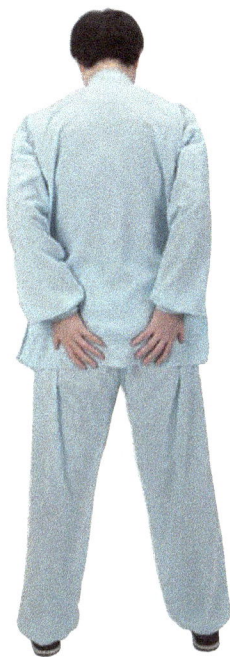

功后动作图25
movements after conclusion 25

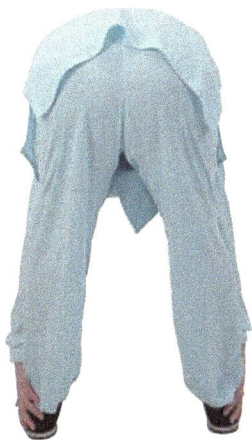

功后动作图26
movements after conclusion 26

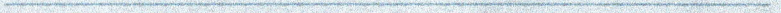

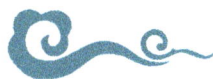

放　松　功　•　*Fang Song Gong* (Relaxation Exercise)

Application

应

用

放松功用于养生保健、疾病的康复，以"松"、"静"为原则，可以根据个人需要，选择放松功法中的任意一种。习练时可整套练习，也可以重点习练松通功中的第一、二步；或三线放松法的第一、二条线路；或重点放松身体的某个部位。每日可练2次，每次15~20分钟，3个月为1个疗程。

Fang Song Gong can benefit health cultivation and aid recovery from illnesses. The essential principle of *Fang Song Gong* is relaxation and tranquil. One can practice the whole set or choose one method. Alternatively, one can focus on movement # 1 and 2 of Song Tong Gong, line # 1 and 2 of Three-Line *Fang Song Gong* or specific body parts. This exercise can be practiced 15-20 minutes each time, twice a day, over 3 months for one course of treatment.

松通法
Relaxing and Unblocking Method

具有调理气机、培补元气的作用。可用于头痛目赤、急躁易怒、腹痛泄泻、夜卧不宁等气机不调的症状；也可用于头晕耳鸣、少气懒言、腰膝酸软等气血不足的症状。高血压、慢性肝炎、失眠多梦、神志不宁、月经不调、遗精滑泻等疾病见上述症状者可参照应用。

This exercise regulates qi activity and supplements yuan-primordial qi. It is indicated for qi-disorder symptoms, including headache, red eyes, irritability, abdominal pain and diarrhea, at restlessness at night. It is also indicated for symptoms due to deficiency of qi and blood, including dizziness, tinnitus, weak breath, reluctance to talk and soreness and weakness in the waist and knees. People with hypertension, chronic hepatitis, insomnia, dream-disturbed sleep, mental unrest, irregular menstruation and nocturnal emissions/spermatorrhea can also practice *Song Tong Gong* if they present with aforementioned symptoms.

三线放松法
Three-line Relaxation Method

具有理气和血、补肾填精的作用。可用于口苦吞酸、胸胁胀满、夜寐不安等气机不调的症状；也可用于头晕耳鸣、腰膝酸软、阳痿早泄等精气不足的症状。高血压、青光眼、慢性疲劳综合征、失眠健忘、两足痿软、腰痛等疾病见上述症状者可参照使用。

This exercise harmonizes qi and blood and supplements kidney essence. It is indicated for qi-disorder symptoms including a bitter taste, acid reflux, fullness and distension in rib-side area and restless at night. It is also indicated for symptoms due to deficiency of yuan-primordial qi including dizziness, tinnitus, soreness and weakness in the waist and knees, impotence and premature ejaculation. People with hypertension, glaucoma, chronic fatigue syndrome, insomnia, poor memory, flaccidity of the feet and low back pain can also practice three-line *Fang Song Gong* if they present with the aforementioned symptoms.

振颤放松法
Body-Shaking/Trembling Relaxation Method

具有疏通经络、益气行血的作用。可用于肢倦身重、不寐、腹胀腹满、心烦胸闷、肩背烦痛等经络不通、气血不和的症状。

慢性疲劳综合征、腰肌劳损、慢性腰背肌筋膜炎、神经衰弱、更年期综合征、颈椎病、超重、脑供血不足等疾病见上述症状者可参照使用。

This exercise unblocks meridians, supplements qi and circulates blood. It is indicated for symptoms due to obstruction of meridians and disharmony between qi and blood, including fatigue and heaviness of the body and limbs, insomnia, abdominal fullness and distension, vexation, chest tightness and shoulder pain. People with chronic fatigue syndrome, lumbar strain, chronic lumbar myofascitis, neurasthenia, menopausal syndrome, cervical spondylosis, overweight and insufficient blood supply to the brain can also practice body-shaking/trembling *Fang Song Gong* if they present with the aforementioned symptoms.

拍打放松法
Tapping Relaxation Method

具有疏通经络、理气活血的作用。可用于胁痛不适、脘腹胀满、肩背烦痛、腰酸背痛等经络不通、气血失调的症状。慢性肝炎、慢性胃炎、消化性溃疡、颈椎病、腰椎病、膝关节炎等疾病见上述症状者可参照应用。

This exercise unblocks meridians, regulates qi and circulates blood. It is indicated for symptoms due to obstruction of meridians and disharmony between qi and blood, including pain and discomfort in the rib-side area, gastric fullness and distension, shoulder pain, lumbar soreness and back pain. People with chronic hepatitis, gastritis, peptic ulcer, cervical spondylosis, lumbar spondylosis and knee osteoarthritis can also practice tapping *Fang Song Gong* if they present with the aforementioned symptoms.

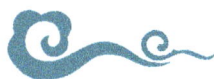

放 松 功　　•　　*Fang Song Gong* (Relaxation Exercise)

The Meridian Charts

经络图

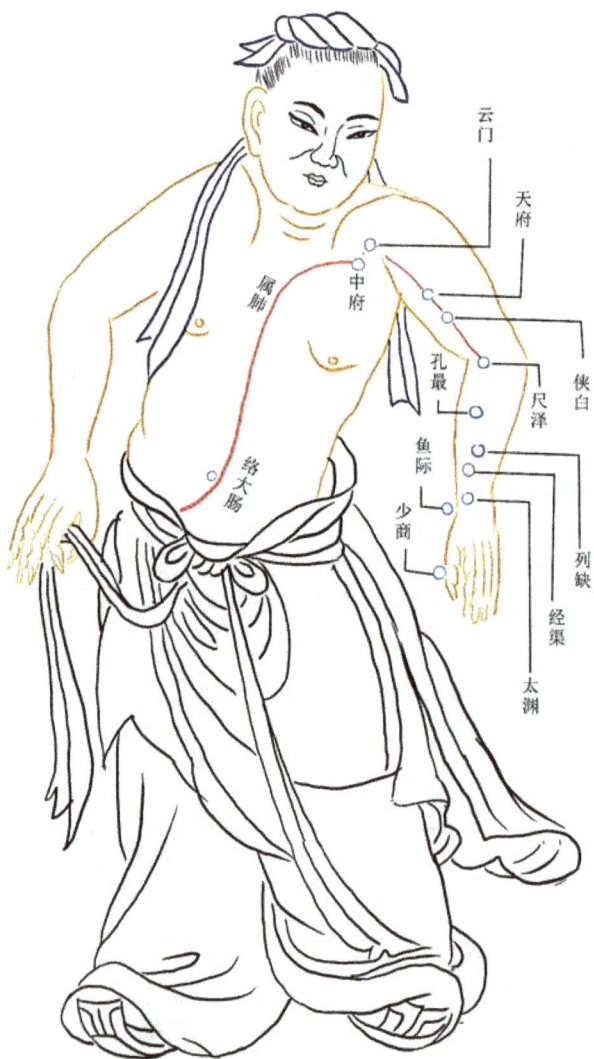

云门
天府
侠白
尺泽
孔最
列缺
经渠
太渊
鱼际
少商
中府
属肺
络大肠

手太阴肺经

Lung Meridian of Hand-Taiyin

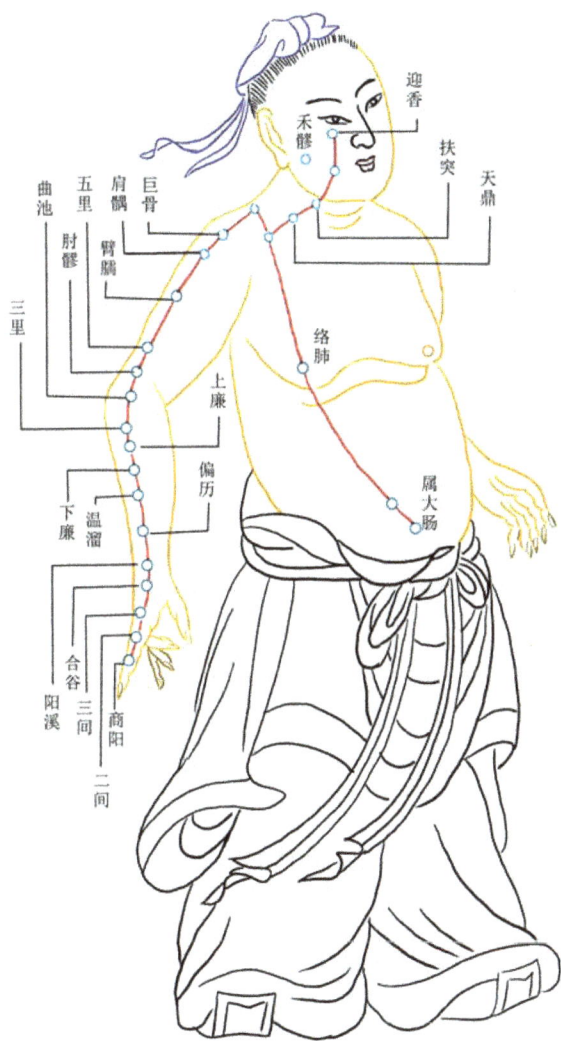

迎香
禾髎
扶突
天鼎
曲池
五里
肩髃
巨骨
臂臑
肘髎
络肺
三里
上廉
偏历
属大肠
下廉
温溜
合谷
三间
阳溪
商阳
二间

手阳明大肠经

Large Intestine Meridian of Hand-Yangming

足阳明胃经

Stomach Meridian of Foot-Yangming

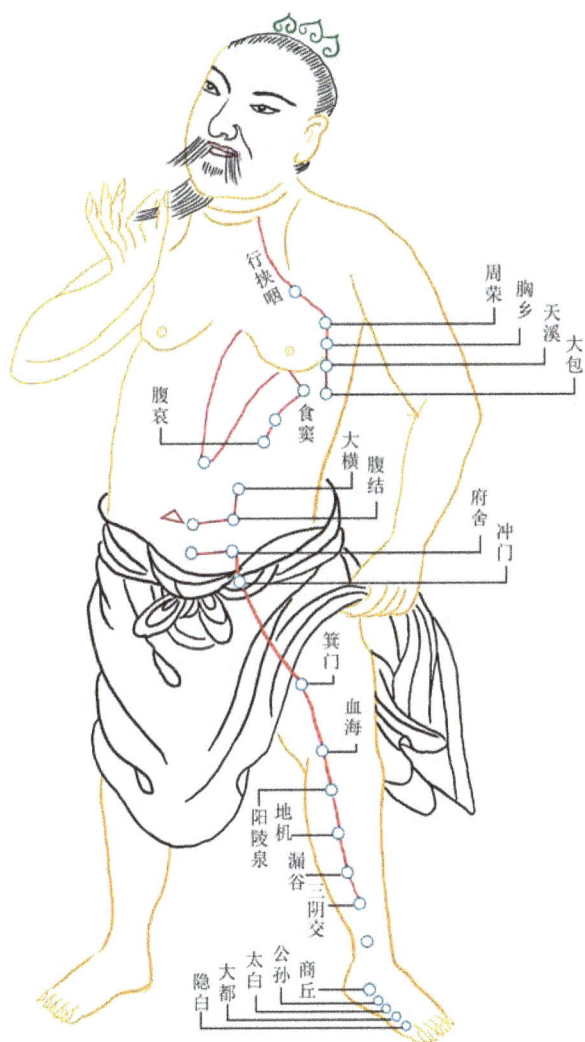

足太阴脾经

Spleen Meridian of Foot-Taiyin

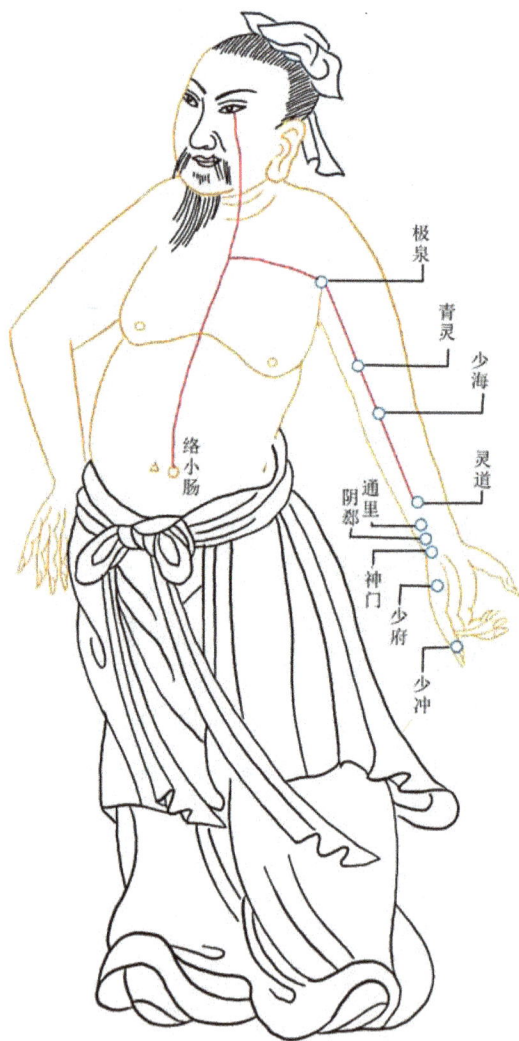

极泉
青灵
少海
灵道
通里
阴郄
神门
少府
少冲
络小肠

手少阴心经

Heart Meridian of Hand-Shaoyin

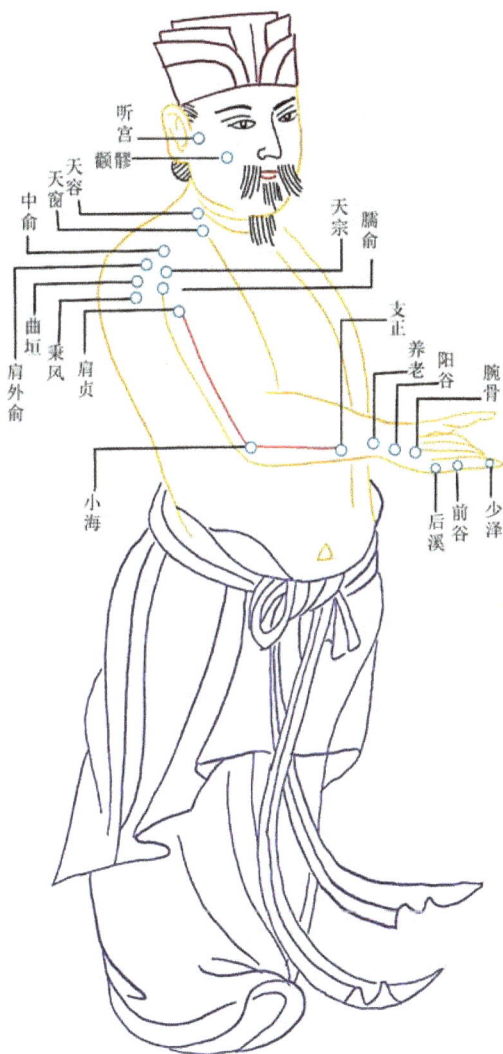

手太阳小肠经

Small Intestine Meridian of Hand-Taiyang

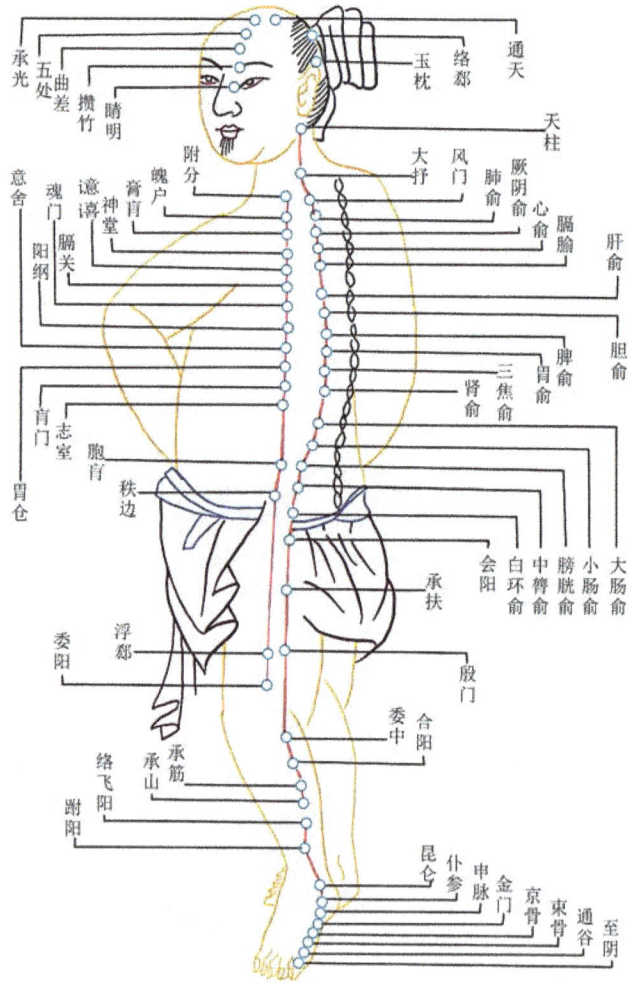

足太阳膀胱经

Bladder Meridian of Foot-Taiyang

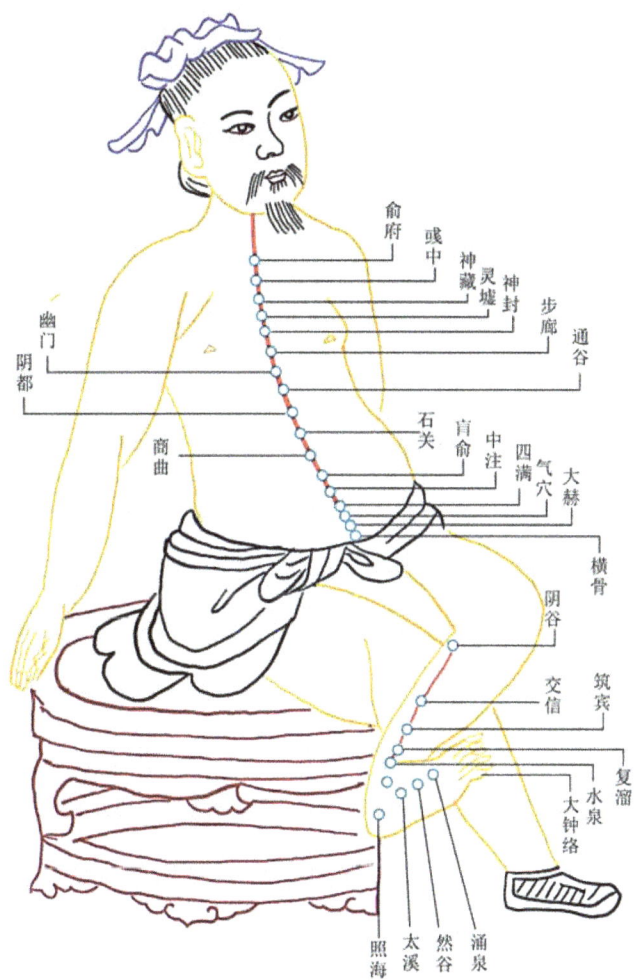

足少阴肾经

Kidney Meridian of Foot-Shaoyin

天泉

出属心包
起胸中
天池

间使
内关
曲泽
郄门

大陵
劳宫

属络三焦

中冲

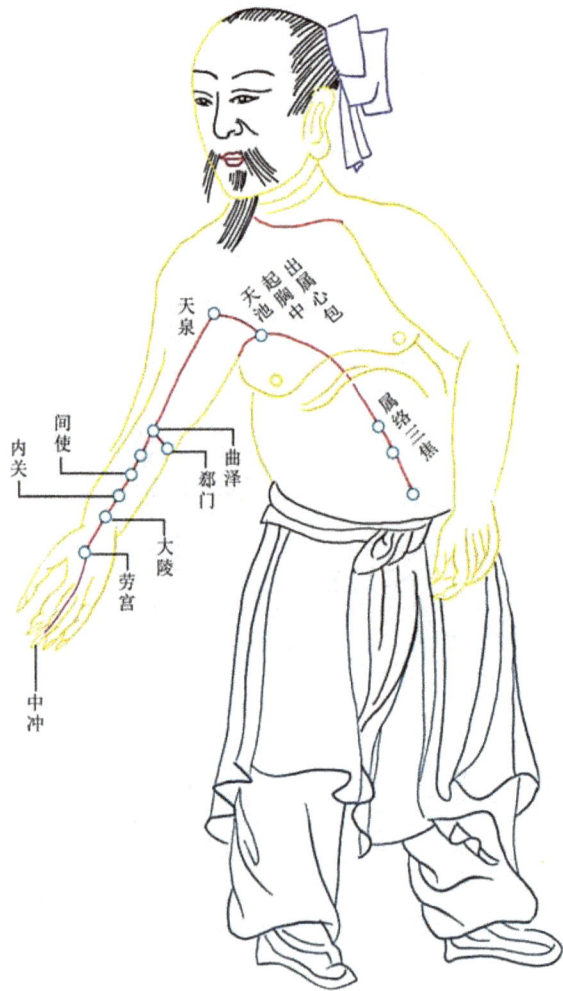

手厥阴心包经

Pericardium Meridian of Hand-Jueyin

丝竹空
和髎
角孙
颅息
耳门
瘛脉
翳风
天牖
天髎
散落心包
臑会
肩髎
消泺
偏属三焦
清冷渊
天井
支沟
四渎
外关
三阳
阳池
会宗
中渚
液门
关冲

手少阳三焦经

Triple Energizer Meridian of Hand-Shaoyang

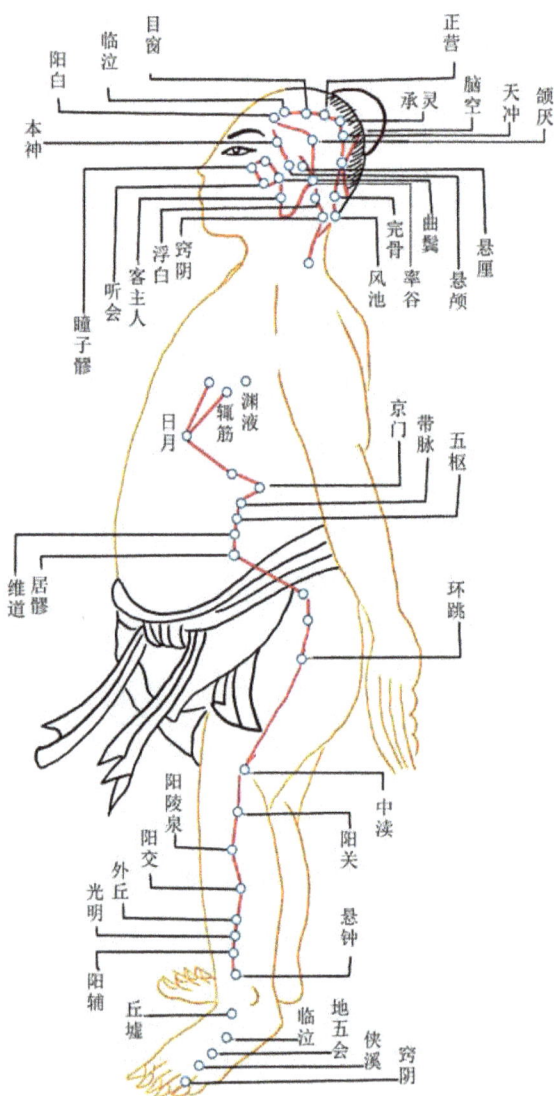

正营
临泣
目窗
脑空
天冲
颔厌
阳白
承灵
本神
曲鬓
率谷
悬厘
悬颅
窍阴
浮白
完骨
客主人
风池
听会
瞳子髎
渊液
辄筋
日月
京门
带脉
五枢
维道
居髎
环跳
中渎
阳陵泉
阳关
阳交
外丘
悬钟
光明
阳辅
丘墟
临泣
地五会
侠溪
窍阴

足少阳胆经

Gallbladder Meridian of Foot-Shaoyang

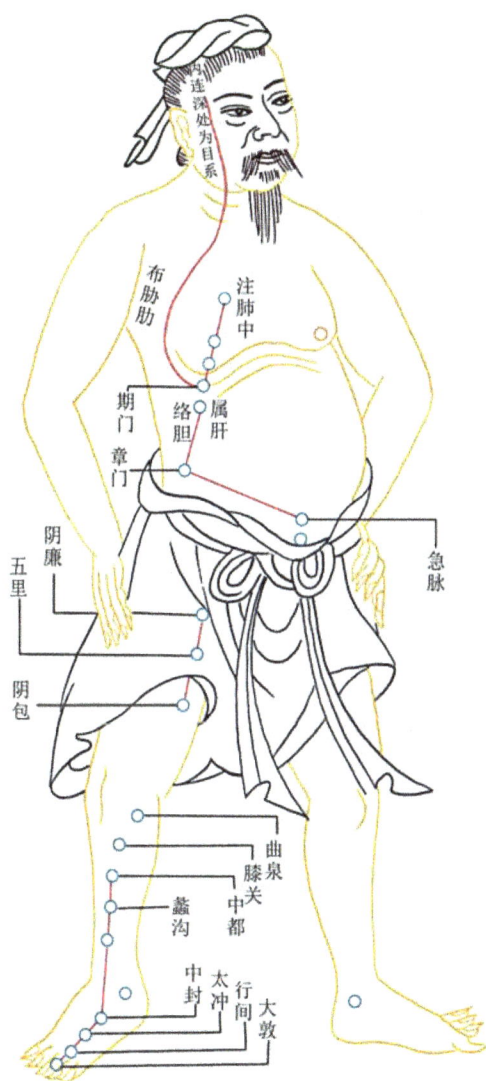

足厥阴肝经

Liver Meridian of Foot-Jueyin

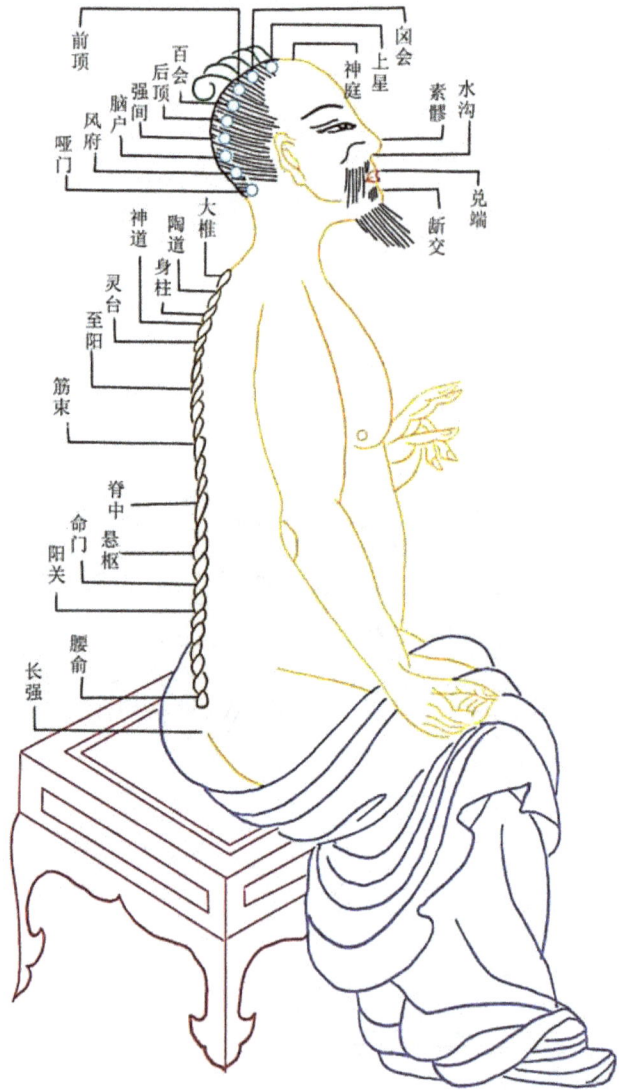

督脉

Governor Vessel (Du)

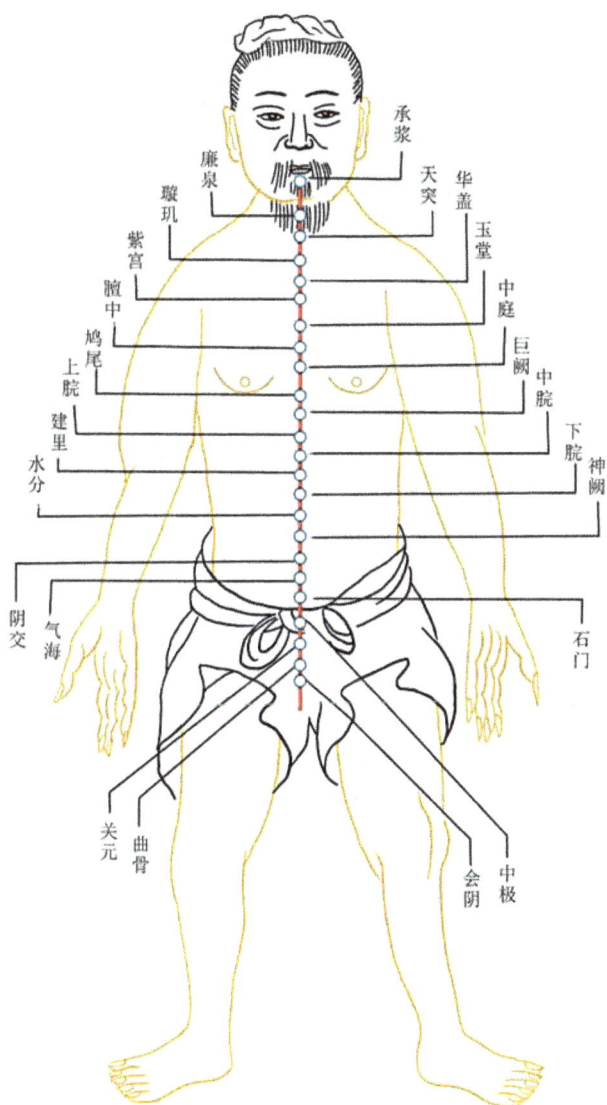

承浆
廉泉
天突
璇玑
华盖
紫宫
玉堂
膻中
中庭
鸠尾
巨阙
上脘
中脘
建里
下脘
水分
神阙
阴交
气海
石门
关元
曲骨
会阴
中极

任脉

Conception Vessel (Ren)

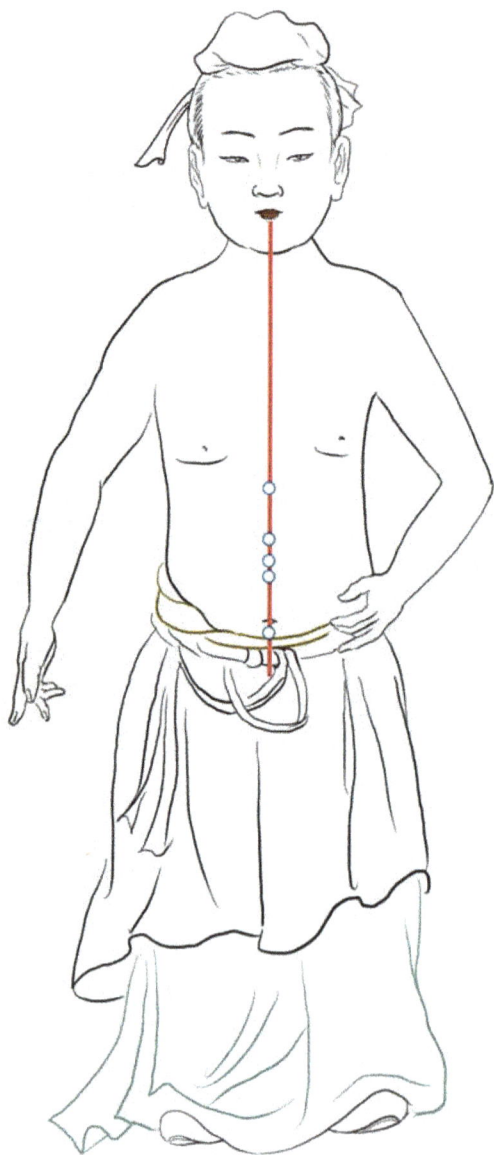

冲脉

Thoroughfare Vessel (Chong)

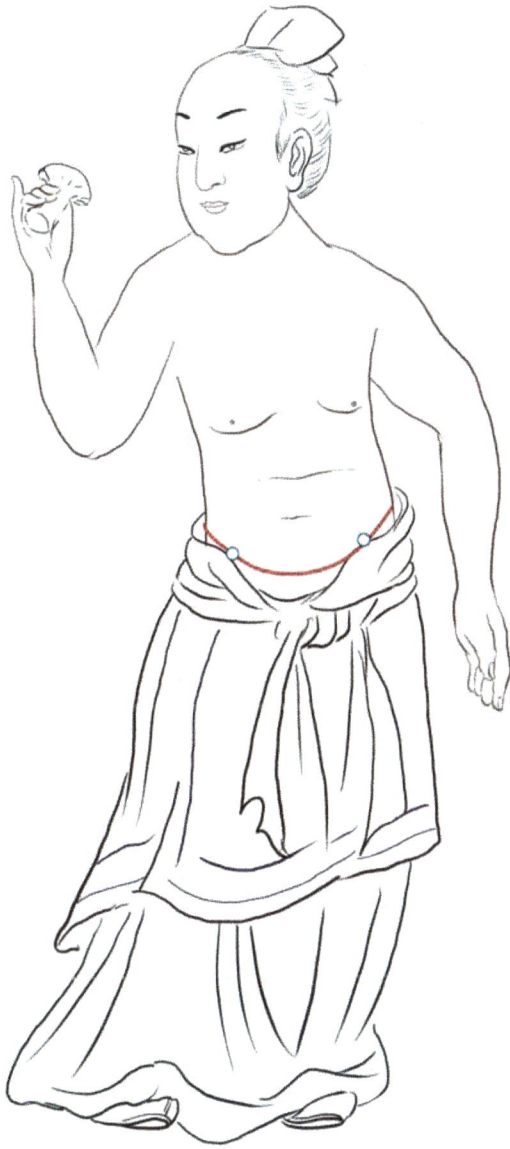

带脉

Belt Vessel (Dai)

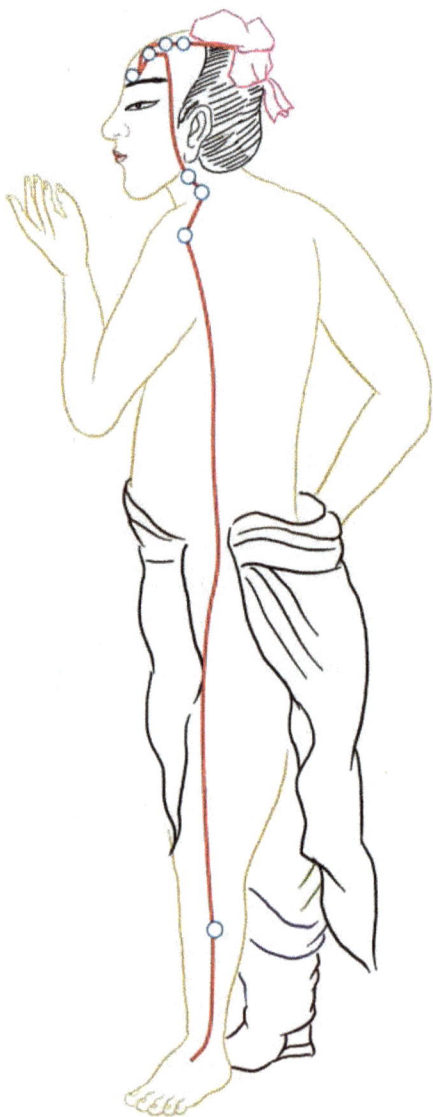

阳维脉

Yang Link Vessel (Yang Wei)

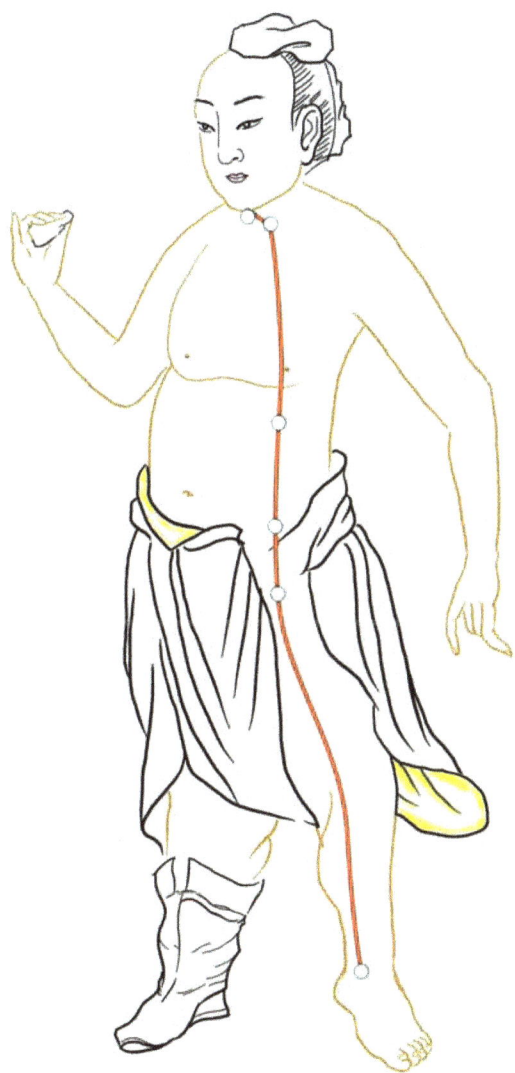

阴维脉

Yin Link Vessel (Yin Wei)

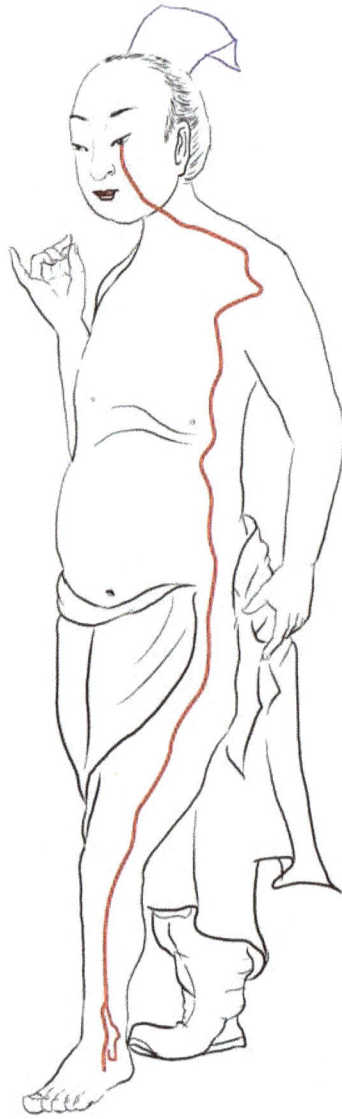

阳蹻脉

Yang Heel Vessel (Yang Qiao)

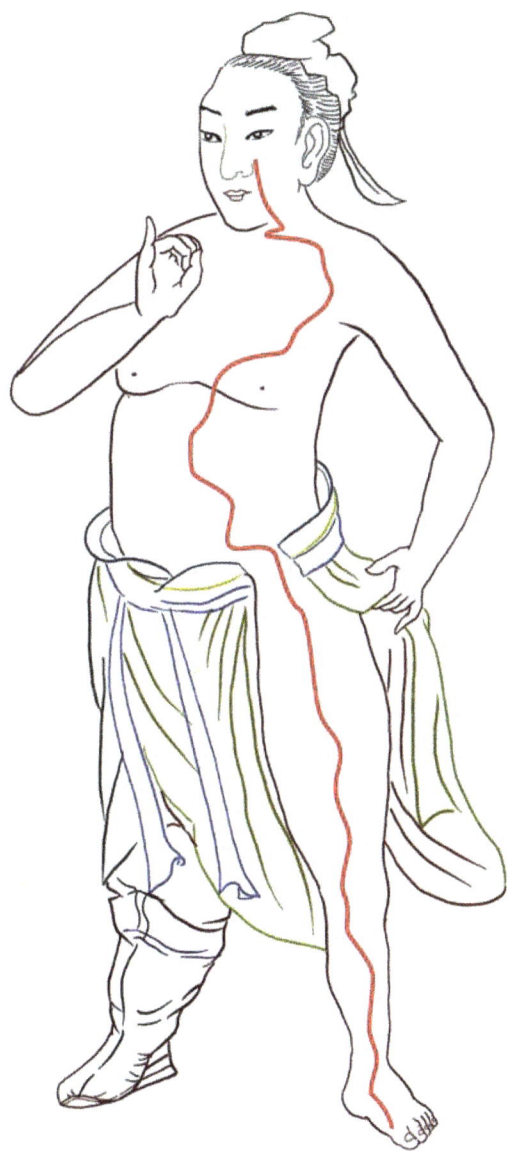

阴蹻脉

Yin Heel Vessel (Yin Qiao)

www.ingramcontent.com/pod-product-compliance
Lightning Source LLC
Chambersburg PA
CBHW081152270326
41930CB00014B/3128